About the Aut

CW01019372

Dr Marilyn Glenville PhD is the UK's leading nutritionist specialising in women's health. She obtained her doctorate from Cambridge University and is a fellow of the Royal Society of Medicine.

Dr Glenville is the former president of the Food and Health Forum at the Royal Society of Medicine and is patron of the Daisy Network, a premature menopause charity.

For more than 40 years, Dr Glenville has studied and practised nutrition, both in the UK and in the USA. She gives lectures and seminars throughout the world and appears regularly on radio and TV.

Dr Glenville has written 16 internationally best-selling books which have sold over one million copies worldwide and have been translated into 20 languages.

The Books Include;

Natural Alternatives to Sugar • *Fat Around the Middle - and How to Get Rid of it* • *Natural Solutions to the Menopause* • *Osteoporosis - How to Prevent, Treat and Reverse it* • *Healthy Eating for the Menopause* • *Natural Solutions to PCOS* • *Natural Solutions to IBS* • *Getting Pregnant Faster* • *Overcoming PMS the Natural Way* • *The Natural Health Bible for Women* • *The Nutritional Health Handbook for Women* • *Natural Solutions for Dementia and Alzheimer's* • *Natural Alternatives to Dieting.*

Dr Glenville has previously won the Best Nutrition Health Writer of the Year Award and has also been awarded a place in the current edition of *Who's Who* of famous people.

Dr Glenville runs clinics in Harley Street in London, Tunbridge Wells in Kent and Dublin and Galway (see *Resources* page at back of book). The Glenville Nutrition Clinic website is www.glenvillenutrition.com.

Acknowledgements

I would like to thank Karen Evennett for helping to make sure that this book is easy to read and to Donna Gambazza for managing the logistics in the background.

I would also like to thank all the nutritionists who work with me in the UK: Helen Ford, Sally Milne, Sharon Pitt and Miki Johnson and those in Ireland, headed by Heather Leeson and Ciara Wright and also Sorcha Molloy in Galway and Lynne Dalton in Dublin. They have a wealth of knowledge and expertise which translates into practical advice that patients can use to transform their health. Thanks go to Audrey Williams who manages the reception in the clinic and was a wonderful support to me, the nutrition team and the patients especially when I was concentrating on writing this book. I also would like to extend my thanks to Birgitta Pain and Caroline Scarborow who seamlessly manage and plan my attendance at the many webinars, exhibitions and conferences l am invited to speak at.

Last but not least, my love goes to my family: Kriss, my husband, and my three children Matt (and his wife Hannah and their children Katie and Jack), Len (and Mel) and Chantell.

Dedication

We all have the power to make the choices to live the best life we can, taking care of mind, body and spirit. I wish you all the best of health dear reader and hope the information in this book helps inspire you to take control of your health and make better and more informed choices.

Natural Solutions To Diabetes -

How To Prevent, Treat, And Reverse Type 2 Diabetes And Prediabetes

Dr Marilyn Glenville PhD

Natural Solutions to Diabetes -
How To Prevent, Treat, and Reverse Type 2 Diabetes and Prediabetes
Dr Marilyn Glenville PhD

First published in the United Kingdom and Ireland in 2022 by Lifestyles Press
14 St John's Road, Tunbridge Wells, Kent TN4 9NP

Conceived, created and designed by Lifestyles Press 2022

Production Manager: Donna Gambazza, Lifestyles Press
Managing Designer: Sian Collins, www.siancollins-designer.com
British Library Cataloguing-in-Publication Data:
A CIP record for this book is available from the British Library

ISBN: 978-1-915292-36-0

Typeset in ITC Garamond BT
Printed in UK

Disclaimer: The contents of this book are for information only and are intended to assist readers in identifying symptoms and conditions they may be experiencing. This book is not intended to be a substitute for taking proper medical advice and should not be relied upon in this way. Always consult a qualified doctor or health practitioner. The author and publisher cannot accept responsibility for illness arising out of the failure to seek medical advice from a doctor.

Contents

Introduction

Whatever your reason for picking up this book – whether you have recently been diagnosed with type 2 diabetes, or you simply want to know more about the condition and how to avoid it – I hope to answer the many questions you are sure to have.

For me, as one of the UK's leading nutritionists, this has been such an important and timely book to write – because type 2 diabetes has now become a worldwide epidemic, and we know that lifestyle and diet have a huge part to play in determining whether you will, or won't, be at risk of developing it.

According to the World Health Organisation (WHO), the number of people with diabetes increased fourfold from 108 million in 1980 to 422 million in 2014. It is now the seventh leading cause of death worldwide and a major cause of blindness, kidney failure, heart attacks, stroke and lower limb amputation.

America's Centers for Disease Control (CDC) states that one in 10 people (that's 34 million) have diabetes and one in three (88 million) have prediabetes. But it's the UK that currently has the fastest growing rate of diabetes in the developing world – with nearly five million people suffering from it: a colossal rise of 450% since 1960. Nine out of 10 of these UK cases are type 2 diabetes. As things stand, every two minutes someone will learn that they have the condition – yet it's thought that nearly another million more people already have type 2 diabetes but are not being diagnosed.

These worrying statistics are only going to get much worse: on top of the millions who have full blown type 2 diabetes in the UK, we have one in three adults with prediabetes– 35.3% – compared to 11.6% in 2003,[1] meaning that they are on their way to developing the disease. Sadly, our grim statistics also include 7,000 young adults and children – some as young as 9 and ten years old; but this is a condition that used to be known as *late onset* or *middle-aged* diabetes.

This is a health crisis of enormous impact, not only for you who are suffering, and your nearest and dearest, but also for our healthcare systems. The NHS spends £10 billion a year on type 2 diabetes, and the condition shockingly results in 7,000 lower leg amputations a year. Being diabetic also makes you at least twice as likely to have a heart attack or stroke.

And yet research proves that this is a lifestyle disease, with the WHO making it clear that a healthy diet, regular physical activity, and maintaining a normal bodyweight can all make the difference to delaying or even preventing it. Indeed, we have seen how an adverse lifestyle has driven the rise in type 2 diabetes in other cultures. For example, China's type 2 diabetes crisis (*the country now has over 100 million people affected by the disease and around half of all Chinese adults are estimated to have pre-diabetes*) is thought to have been driven by the introduction of a more Westernised diet (together with a reduction in physical activity and a rise in psychosocial stress, resulting in an increase in rates of obesity.[2]

Elsewhere, in Mexico, type 2 diabetes became a crisis in 2006. Already the country's leading cause of death, cases had doubled in six years. With 75,000 amputations a year caused by diabetes and a major obesity crisis not only in adults but also in children (between 1999 and 2006 obesity rose by 40% in children 5-11), the Mexican government decided to put a 10% tax on soft drinks in 2014. This has resulted in a 10% decrease in soft drink consumption and a revenue of 1.9 billion pesos. It could be argued that if they collected so much revenue then people did not stop buying soft drinks, they just paid more for them. But in 2014 the sales of taxed drinks fell by six per cent, and sales of bottled water rose by four per cent.

Scientists predict that, over a 10 year period, this tax will have resulted in nearly 200,000 fewer cases of type 2 diabetes, along with 20,000 fewer strokes and heart attacks.

How This Book Can Help You

You **need** to read this book if you have been diagnosed with type 2 diabetes. Not only do you need to know more about what your diagnosis means, and how it affects your body and your long-term health – but, most importantly, you also need to know what you can do about it. Maybe you have just been diagnosed and are keen to know what you can do to help yourself while you wait to be prescribed medication. Or you may already be on medication for your diabetes and want to know what you should do alongside the medication, with a view to being able to reduce or eventually stop taking the drugs.

You **should** also read this book if you have a family history of type 2 diabetes and are worried that you are going to go down the same path, and want to know how to avoid that fate.

But, above all, you **MUST** read this book if you have been diagnosed with prediabetes. You are literally at a crossroads with your health right now. If you do nothing, you will develop full-blown type 2 diabetes within a few years – but, by taking action, you could stop it in its tracks, and my methods really can help.

Everything I recommend in this book is natural, safe and will only boost your general health – wouldn't it be a wonderful bonus if it reversed your type 2 diabetes too? And, let's face it; you've got nothing to lose by trying.

Yes, you'll need to be committed. But believe me, it will be SO worth it!

The aim of this book is to give you back control over your body and to let you know that you do not have to 'put up' with type 2 diabetes for one day longer. I hope you enjoy it, and that it informs and inspires you.

PART 1

UNDERSTANDING DIABETES

Chapter 1

What is diabetes?

"All types of diabetes involve higher than normal levels of glucose (sugar) in the blood."

The focus of this book is on prediabetes and type 2 diabetes. However, you will know that there are other forms of diabetes too – type 1, type 3 and gestational diabetes. Although the causes of these different forms vary greatly, all types of diabetes involve higher than normal levels of glucose (sugar) in the blood. It may help to put your own condition in perspective if we take a brief look at the other forms of diabetes.

Type 1 Diabetes

Type 1 diabetes is often diagnosed in childhood – although some people can be diagnosed later in life. It is classed as an auto-immune disease because your own immune system kills the cells (beta-cells) in the pancreas that produce insulin, the hormone that enables vital energy from your food to reach your cells. Without any naturally-occurring insulin, the only way to thrive and survive is to use insulin injections (or an insulin pump) – and, having been diagnosed with type 1, you will need to do this for the rest of your life.

The important tell-tale signs of type 1 diabetes are:

- Feeling very thirsty
- Peeing more than usual, particularly at night
- Feeling very tired
- Losing weight without trying
- Thrush that keeps coming back

- Blurred vision

- Cuts and grazes that are not healing

You should see your doctor if you are getting any of these symptoms. It's worth knowing that they can come on quite suddenly.

Type 2 Diabetes

Type 2 diabetes is often called middle-aged onset diabetes, because it usually develops later in life – although we are now, sadly, seeing an increasing number of children with the disorder. It is often associated with being overweight.

Whereas with type 1 diabetes your pancreas is unable to produce the insulin you need in order to survive, if you have type 2 diabetes, your pancreas continues to produce insulin, but your body stops responding to it. This is known as insulin resistance, and means the normal process of insulin helping glucose (sugar) enter your cells to provide energy is not working. I will discuss insulin resistance in more detail in Chapter 2.

The first line of treatment in type 2 diabetes is with insulin sensitising medication (for example metformin). This increases your cells' sensitivity to insulin so that they take in more glucose (sugar) and, therefore, lower the amount of glucose (sugar) accumulating in your blood. But if, despite these drugs and due to insulin resistance, your pancreas keeps having to overwork, then its insulin-producing beta cells may fail and, like someone with type 1 diabetes, you may end up having to use insulin injections or a pump.

You should see your doctor to be tested for type 2 diabetes if you have any of the following symptoms:

- Increased thirst

- Frequent urination

- Fatigue

- Blurred vision

Prediabetes

There is now a name for the stage that precedes full blown type 2 diabetes: 'prediabetes'. Discovering you have prediabetes may be upsetting, but it can also be a very useful diagnosis – in fact, for many people I have seen in my clinic, it has been just the wake-up call they needed. They are shocked by the diagnosis but they realise that they are now at a crossroads. One road will lead to full blown type 2 diabetes in just a few short years – and they will embark on this daunting trajectory if they don't take action to improve their lifestyle. Alternatively, they can take another route, which will help them to reverse their poor health, not only dodging the diabetes bullet but also gaining the chance to enjoy good health for years to come – because prediabetes is linked to many other very serious conditions too.

There are not many clear-cut symptoms relating to prediabetes, however you might see darkened skin on certain areas of your body – a condition known as *acanthosis nigricans*. This is often found between your elbow and shoulder and, at first, you might think your skin is just dirty. You can also develop skin tags (*acrochordons*), floppy bits of skin that can grow anywhere but are most commonly found on the neck, underarms and eyelids. Skin tags don't necessarily indicate prediabetes, but they can show that your blood sugar is not as balanced as it should be.

Regardless of any symptoms, it is suggested that you are checked for prediabetes if you are overweight, with a BMI of over 25, and/or you are over the age of 45.

Testing is especially important if you also have any of these other risk factors:

- You have a strong family history risk of type 2 diabetes
- You're physically inactive
- You have a history of gestational diabetes or have ever given birth to a baby weighing more than nine pounds (4kg)
- You have, or have had, PCOS (polycystic ovary syndrome)
- You have high triglycerides or low 'good' HDL cholesterol

Type 2 diabetes, and prediabetes, are diagnosed with a blood test and I will explain more about testing later in the book.

Gestational Diabetes

This is a form of diabetes which typically starts during pregnancy but usually disappears once you have given birth. Unfortunately, though, half of all women who develop gestational diabetes go on to develop full blown type 2 diabetes 10 to 15 years later.

Gestational diabetes can put you more at risk of developing high blood pressure during the pregnancy. It also increases your chance of needing a caesarean section, and makes it very likely that you would give birth to a much larger baby (over 9lbs or 4kg) as the higher glucose (sugar) levels in your blood make the baby grow bigger.

Type 3 Diabetes

Like the other cells elsewhere in your body, those in your brain can become insulin resistant – meaning that your brain can become deprived of the energy that the neurons need in order to function healthily. This can cause slower thinking, brain fog, and loss of focus and concentration – and, as a result of insulin resistance, people with type 2 diabetes are also about 50 to 60% more likely than average to develop Alzheimer's.[3] This research has led to a new diagnosis of type 3 diabetes, specifically linked to Alzheimer's.

The good news is that treating type 2 diabetes with insulin sensitisers can improve brain function and also slow the rate of cognitive decline in Alzheimer's. The same researchers have said that many type 2 diabetics have deposits of a protein (amyloid beta) in their pancreas which is similar to that found in the brain with Alzheimer's – so it may be possible to prevent and slow down both diseases simultaneously as the cause is, effectively, the same.

In addition to type 3 diabetes, it's important to know that insulin resistance is thought to trigger inflammation in the brain and vascular changes (changes in blood vessels) that could cause micro strokes, known as TIAs (transient ischaemic attacks).

Metabolic Syndrome

I want to say a few words about metabolic syndrome here. Although separate to type 2 diabetes, it is a condition that – as a diabetic, or prediabetic – you really need to be aware of, because type 2 diabetes is a contributory factor, and many people who have type 2 diabetes also have the additional symptoms that, clustered together with your high blood sugar, form metabolic syndrome. These symptoms are: high cholesterol, high triglycerides, high blood pressure and a larger waist circumference.

Having this cluster of problems – which is very common and thought to affect up to one in three adults over the age of 50 – puts you at higher risk of heart disease and stroke, and even the threat of metabolic syndrome should be even more of a wake-up call for your health than prediabetes – because lifestyle factors have such a big part to play. High LDL ("bad") cholesterol, high triglycerides, high blood sugar and high blood pressure very often go hand-in-hand with being overweight, eating unhealthily and taking too little exercise. These are all things that you can do something about, when you know how (and I will show you). There are, of course, medical solutions to the symptoms of metabolic syndrome but, even alongside these, it is absolutely vital to address your lifestyle choices too.

The reason I am so passionate about lifestyle is that it puts you in control of your health and, with a condition like metabolic syndrome, it is so easy to lose that control.

Just think about it: you could be seeing a cardiologist who is concerned about your high cholesterol levels, while also seeing an endocrinologist for your type 2 diabetes. You have the same blood and hormones passing through every system in your body, and it is easy to see that you could have an underlying cause that may be affecting every organ – but, by seeing separate doctors for these separate issues, it's possible that no-one is considering the overall picture. As a result, you could easily end up on different drugs for each symptom, many of which will then cause side effects needing further drugs… But there are very often lifestyle changes you can make to address the underlying roots of all your problems and the aim of this book is to show you how to make these changes – and transform your health for the better.

Drugs v Lifestyle

Imagine your health as a tree, with various problems attached to different branches. For example, you might have high cholesterol, high blood pressure, weight gain, blood sugar imbalances and maybe other symptoms such as lack of energy, mood swings, headaches and digestive problems.

All of these could be treated separately, so you are given statins for the high cholesterol, antihypertensive medication for the high blood pressure, metformin for the blood sugar problems, antidepressants for your low mood and painkillers for your headaches. But each medication can have side effects – which are bad enough that you need further drugs to help you cope with them.

A good example of this – and something you may not know – is that the statins you may be given to lower your cholesterol can actually increase your risk of type 2 diabetes, possibly by up to 46%![4] The higher the dose of the statins, the higher your risk.

So, the suggestion is that people who are on statins should offset their risk of diabetes by also taking the diabetes drug glyburide[5].

But glyburide carries its own side effects. The most common are heartburn and nausea, so you may then be prescribed antacids or proton pump inhibitors (PPIs) to stop these side effects. But the PPIs increase the risk of Alzheimer's and osteoporosis which will, in turn, need medication… And so it goes on…!

Beneath this tree, with its many branches of symptoms, are the roots which feed and nourish it. The nourishment the tree gets determines how well the leaves on the branches grow and how

---

it blossoms. It's clear that in, order to affect the symptoms that appear on your branches, you need to do some work on the roots.

That is the aim of this book: to show you how to nourish the underlying root cause of your health problem. And then, once your tree is healthy, it will only need a simple maintenance programme to keep it that way.

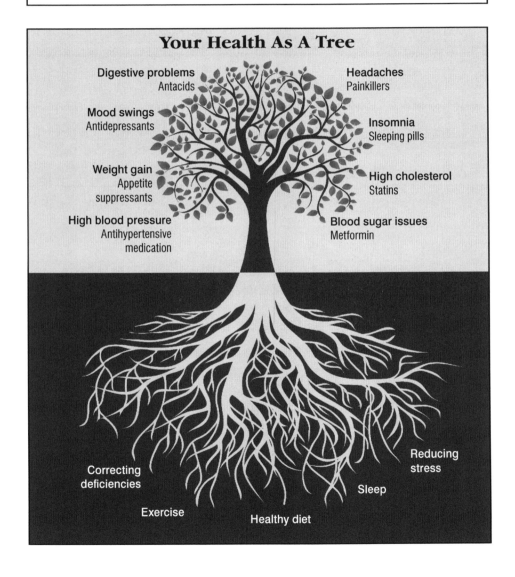

Your Health As A Tree

Digestive problems
Antacids

Headaches
Painkillers

Mood swings
Antidepressants

Insomnia
Sleeping pills

Weight gain
Appetite
suppressants

High cholesterol
Statins

High blood pressure
Antihypertensive
medication

Blood sugar issues
Metformin

Reducing
stress

Correcting
deficiencies

Sleep

Exercise

Healthy diet

Chapter 2

Diet, digestion and diabetes

"Foods that are digested very quickly result in much higher levels of glucose (sugar) in your blood, and this will require more insulin to be released by your pancreas."

It is helpful to know what is happening in your body with type 2 diabetes because, the more you understand, the easier it will be to make changes and see how they are benefiting your health. Your increased knowledge and understanding will also help to keep you motivated when you might have days where you might not be eating so well.

In Chapter 1, I touched on the fact that all types of diabetes involve high levels of glucose (sugar) in your blood – and this is important because, when your blood sugar level is too high for too long, it can lead to very serious health problems including kidney damage, stroke, heart disease, nerve, eye and skin damage.

But, go back a step, and diabetes is fundamentally about insulin.

Produced by your pancreas, insulin is the hormone that helps to divert glucose (sugar) out of your blood and into your muscles to give you energy. If something goes wrong with this process, and – as in type 2 diabetes – your body is unable to use insulin in the normal way, you will not be able to get the energy you need from your food, and, because glucose is not leaving your bloodstream in the way that it should, you will also end up with high blood glucose (sugar).

So, what *should* be happening when your body is functioning healthily?

Let's start by looking at what happens when you eat.

Your meal or snack is broken down by digestion into glucose (sugar) and absorbed through the walls of your small intestine into your blood – and it's perfectly natural to have a higher level of glucose in your blood straight after a meal. Your pancreas then releases insulin to move the glucose (sugar) out of your blood and into your cells to be used for energy. If you have taken in more glucose or sugar than your body needs for energy, the excess will be changed into glycogen and stored in your liver and muscles to be used later. The glucose level in your blood should then return to a normal level – because, under normal circumstances, your body has a brilliant balancing mechanism for keeping your blood sugar in balance: when your blood sugar level rises too high, your body produces more insulin to balance it. If your blood sugar level is too low, the hormones adrenaline and cortisol are released from the adrenal glands and they stimulate the production of another hormone, glucagon (also from the pancreas). Glucagon works in the opposite way to insulin and increases blood glucose by encouraging the liver to turn some of its glycogen stores into glucose.

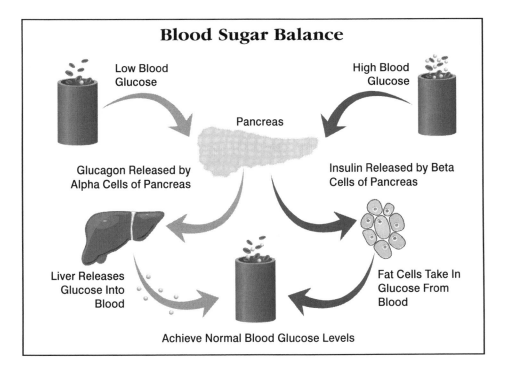

Blood Sugar Balance

Low Blood Glucose

High Blood Glucose

Pancreas

Glucagon Released by Alpha Cells of Pancreas

Insulin Released by Beta Cells of Pancreas

Liver Releases Glucose Into Blood

Fat Cells Take In Glucose From Blood

Achieve Normal Blood Glucose Levels

So far, so good. But do remember that not all foods are digested at the same speed. Anything high in sugar or refined carbohydrates, like white pasta and bread, will be digested very quickly, resulting in much higher levels of glucose (sugar) in your blood which, in turn, will require more insulin to be released by your pancreas. It is released to direct energy from your food to your cells, with the excess going into storage in the form of glycogen. But there is a limit to how much excess sugar can be stored as glycogen – and what cannot be usefully stored in this way will, instead, be stored as fat. In fact, you could think of insulin as the 'fat storing hormone' of your body – and the more insulin you produce the more your food is likely to be stored as fat.

Unfortunately, when your insulin levels are high, your body doesn't use fat for fuel; it uses the glucose in your blood instead. So, when insulin is being produced, you won't lose weight; instead your body will cling on to your fat stores.

This matters because, as I mentioned in chapter 1, being overweight is one of the factors that can contribute (along with type 2 diabetes, high cholesterol and high blood pressure) to you developing metabolic syndrome.

But carrying too much fat on your body (and particularly if it is around your middle) also increases your risk of developing insulin resistance – especially if you are also physically inactive. This is because excess fat around the middle produces inflammatory substances, and it is thought that these substances play a role in causing insulin resistance. (Meanwhile, physical activity is thought to help regulate blood sugar levels, reducing the risk of insulin resistance.)

For the record, a waist measurement of 37 inches (94 cm) or more for men, or 31.5 inches (80 cm) or more for women is linked to insulin resistance, *even if you have a normal body weight or BMI.*

A further problem, if your body fat percentage is raised too high, is that you can also become *leptin resistant*. This means that your body will not register the effects of this hormone – whose role is to regulate your appetite by letting you know when you are full and can stop eating. Consequently, you will end up feeling less satisfied, and may inadvertently overeat.

Another hormone that impacts on leptin is cortisol. This is the stress hormone that is released along with another stress hormone, adrenaline, when your blood sugar drops and one of its actions is to prevent leptin from decreasing your appetite.

Over the next chapters of this book I will show you how you can manage the hormones that control your weight and diabetes risk. Your journey to a healthier you has just begun!

Understanding Your Pancreas

Your pancreas plays a critical role in diabetes. This long, flat gland, about the size of your hand, sits behind your stomach. It produces insulin along with a number of other hormones including glucagon, somatostatin, gastrin, amylin and pancreatic polypeptide. It also plays a part in your digestive system – neutralising stomach acid with bicarbonate from the pancreatic juice it secretes, and producing digestive enzymes which break down fats (the enzyme lipase), protein (the enzyme protease) and carbohydrates (the enzyme amylase).

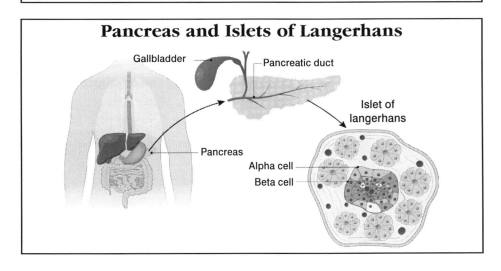

Pancreas and Islets of Langerhans

The Role Of Insulin

Your pancreas has cells called the Islets of Langerhans (named after the German pathologist who discovered them). These include alpha cells, which produce glucagon, and beta cells, which make insulin.

Throughout your body, insulin receptors on your cells act like locks, waiting for insulin (the key) to open them so that glucose (sugar) from your bloodstream can move in. Your cells can then use the glucose for energy and your blood glucose level (or blood sugar level) is lowered.

However, if you continue with an unhealthy diet and lifestyle, you can become insulin resistant. The insulin receptors do not open in response to insulin and the glucose from your blood is not moved into your cells. This means you are not getting the energy you need from your food and you also end up with high blood glucose (sugar).

Insulin Resistance

I talked about insulin resistance earlier because it is an important aspect of what is happening in type 2 diabetes. As I have mentioned elsewhere, it is not that you are producing too little insulin from the pancreas but that your body cannot use it. Sometimes you may even be producing too much insulin but still your body cannot use it. When the cells in your muscles, fat and liver can't take up the sugar (glucose) from your blood, your pancreas makes more insulin to try and overcome this. If your pancreas keeps receiving information that blood glucose is too high, then it will try to produce even more insulin. But the more insulin that is produced the less effective it becomes and the more resistant to insulin your cells will be.

Having too high levels of insulin also has other consequences. Remember that insulin is your fat-storing hormone and promotes the formation of fat (lipogenesis), which, of course, causes you to gain weight. As you will read on pages 68-70, high levels of insulin also increase your risk of cancer.

It is thought that testing your fasting insulin levels could be an effective way to establish whether you have insulin resistance, even if you don't have diabetes, and this could be used as a way to identify people who might go on to develop type 2 diabetes.[6] (Information about testing insulin is mentioned in Chapter 26.)

Producing insulin that your body cannot use also has a knock-on effect on other hormones, and one of these is to block the production of leptin – your appetite control hormone. Leptin is produced by your fat cells and its job is to warn you that you have had enough to eat – it's responsible for that satisfied feeling. So, you might think that the more fat you have, the better the effect would be, as you would be producing even more leptin – but, in fact, as we've seen above, the reverse is true.

Chapter 3

Understanding your risks

"Knowing you are at risk is an extra reason to optimise your health."

While many of the risk factors – your age, race, gender and genes – cannot be avoided, these risks do not make the eventual onset of diabetes an inevitability and they are no reason to give up on the things that you *can* change, such as your diet and how active you are. Instead, if you know that your gender and genes are against you, see this as an extra reason to optimise your health with the lifestyle measures that I will discuss in detail in later chapters.

The main underlying risk factors that I will outline here are: weight, race, gender, age, family history, genes and Polycystic Ovary Syndrome (PCOS).

1. Your Weight

Research shows that if you are obese (with a BMI of 30 or above), you are 80 times more likely to develop type 2 diabetes than those with a BMI of less than 22.[7]

• Body Mass Index (BMI)

The most commonly accepted measure of whether or not you are overweight is known as the Body Mass Index (BMI). This is the ratio of your height to your weight and is calculated by dividing your weight in kilograms by the square of your height in metres. For example, if your weight is 63.5kg (10 stone) and your height is 1.68m (5ft 6in), your BMI will be 63.5 ÷ 1.68 x 1.68 = 22.5. (There are many easy-to-use BMI calculators online if you don't fancy doing the maths yourself.)

This result of this calculation puts you into a certain weight category:

Under 20	=	underweight
20–25	=	normal weight
25–30	=	overweight
30–40	=	obese
Over 40	=	dangerously obese

But are you really overweight, or – more importantly – could you be overfat?

The drawback of the BMI as a measure is that it cannot allow for variations in fat, bone, organs and muscle. And, as muscle is heavier than fat, so the BMI of a 'well-built', extremely fit person might be as high as that of an unfit, rather fat person. Similarly, it is quite possible to be overfat and yet not overweight, and to register, therefore, with a relatively low BMI. But remember – that does *not* mean you're safe and healthy!

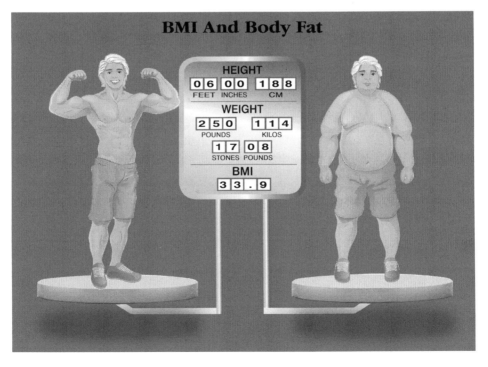

• How Much Fat Are You Carrying And Where Are You Carrying It?

You can measure your body fat percentage with a body composition machine (I've always found Tanita a good make) and nowadays they are often the size of a set of bathroom scales, and a similar price too. An electric current is passed (painlessly) though your body and the machine measures how long it takes for the current to go from one foot to the other. Muscle is a much better conductor of electricity than fatty tissue so, the more muscular you are, the quicker the current will pass. The more fat you have, the slower the current. The speed is then converted into a 'fat percentage' score.

Women naturally carry more fat than men, but both genders' percentage of fat will usually increase with age, as we become less active and lose muscle. For women, a healthy fat percentage is between 21 and 36% and for men 12 and 25%.

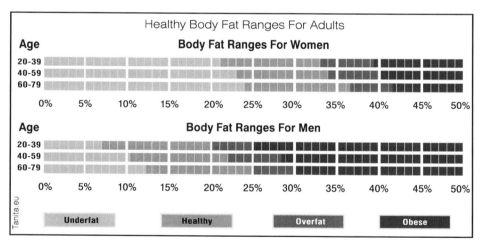

But, *where* your fat is situated can make all the difference to your health and your risk of type 2 diabetes – and, with this in mind, another important way to check your risk is to measure your waist-to-hip ratio.

Take a tape measure and compare your waist measurement (about an inch above your belly button) with your hip measurement (at the widest point). Divide the waist figure by the hip figure to get your waist-to-hip ratio.

For example, 86cm (34in) (waist) ÷ 94cm (37in) (hip) = 0.9. Anything over 0.8 for a woman is unhealthy (apple shaped), while men are unhealthy with a waist-to-hip ratio over 9.5.

You can also just measure your waist circumference. You are at risk of type 2 diabetes if, as a woman, your waist measures 31.5in (80cm) or more and, for a man, 37in (94cm) or more. For men of South Asian origin, it is 35in (89cm) or more, though for women it is still 31.5in (80cm) or more.

Unfortunately, if you are of South Asian origin, you can be more genetically predisposed to type 2 diabetes and up to six times more likely to develop it than people of Western or European origin.

Waist measurement is an easy indicator of potential problems but one that is often overlooked by the medical profession, even though your weight and height are usually measured during health checks! I am intrigued by the fact that such an important indicator is overlooked, and have come across one comment, in a medical journal, stating that 'many physicians are more comfortable offering a plasma insulin level and prescribing insulin-sensitising medications than measuring a waist circumference and discussing diet and physical activity.'[8] This is such a shame – and a missed opportunity. Instead of giving their patients the wherewithal to take control of their own health, many find it quicker and easier to simply write a prescription – even knowing that, as we've seen in the last chapter, one drug may soon lead to another and another and another as the doctor tries to head off a litany of potential side effects.

I find it very concerning that doctors are reluctant to measure waist circumference when it is such a useful measure. There are many reasons why their patients may be overeating and under-exercising and some of these can be extremely complex and difficult for a time-starved doctor to tackle. But it has also been suggested that doctors and nurses shy away from measuring patients' waists because they don't have protocols for doing this consistently and correctly – and they also that patients might feel embarrassed about having their waist measured.[9] I am not sure how measuring a person's waist can be more embarrassing than a cervical smear or prostate test! The same research suggests that lack of time and extra workload could be obstacles – having a conversation about diet and lifestyle is often time-consuming and complicated - but, interestingly, the researchers said that the patients generally raised few barriers to having their waists measured, especially after an explanation was given as to why it was important for them.

And then comes the issue about fat-shaming and how health care professionals need to approach the issue of weight (and waist circumference) without causing offence. It is, sadly, not unknown for people to even feel insulted by the suggestion that they could have diabetes and should be tested. Yes, pride and embarrassment can sometimes prevent patients from getting the help they need – and knowing this can also stop their doctors from offering it!

Healthcare professionals need to be able to warn their patients of the dangers to their health. I have found in my clinics, over the 35 years that I have been in practice, that the best way to approach this is without criticism, guilt or fault on the part of the person but to says words along the line that 'we need to do something about this and I can help you'. The person does want help, and that is why they have come to see me, and are asking for a solution but need support and guidance in order to achieve their goals. I also think that, unfortunately, doctors get very little in the way of nutritional education over their five or more years in medical school. As such, they don't always know what is the best advice to give and, therefore, avoid it.

• Fat Around Your Middle

The process that drives weight to gather around your middle is controlled by the hormones insulin and cortisol. The message sent to your body from high insulin levels as your blood sugar rises is to store your food as fat. Then again, when your blood sugar drops, cortisol is released and the message this hormone sends out is more of the same: store that fat around your middle.

In evolutionary terms, this is a protective mechanism and, when you understand the underlying biology, you can see why your body would want to store fat here – because, for your caveman ancestors, having a store of fat in times of stress was essential, providing them with the instant fuel they needed for fight or flight. The problem now is that stress hormones still cause fat to store around our middles for these emergency situations – even when we will not be required to flee in a hurry, or fight off a woolly mammoth or sabre tooth tiger! Your body doesn't care that you're stressed because you're up against a work deadline or your washing machine has broken down. It will still release the same stress hormones that trigger the cascade of actions that result in that fat around your middle.

Nobody likes the look of a wodge of weight sitting around the middle and it's a source of great misery to many people, particularly women. Clothes don't fit properly or look as good and *'I look pregnant'* is a common complaint from my patients. But, vanity aside, having fat around your middle increases your risk of becoming insulin resistant, which can lead to type 2 diabetes. This is because fat around your middle is metabolically active (compared to the inactive fat on your hips). As such, it operates like an endocrine gland producing a number of compounds that can affect your health. It increases your risk of type 2 diabetes because it releases a protein called retinol-binding protein 4 (RBP4) which increases resistance to insulin. But it also increases your risk of heart disease, high blood pressure, stroke, cancer (especially breast cancer) and Alzheimer's. For example, recent research has shown that women who quickly gain belly fat during menopause could be at a greater risk of heart disease. In a study at the University of Pittsburgh, scientists repeatedly measured the fat around the organs (visceral fat) of women participants using a CT scan and also used ultrasound to look at the thickness of the internal carotid artery (an early indicator of heart disease). The results were astonishing. For every 20% increase in belly fat, the thickness of the carotid artery increased by two per cent irrespective of overall weight, BMI or any other risk factors for heart disease. The study's authors recommend measuring belly fat as well as looking at weight and BMI for a more accurate indication of heart disease risk.[10]

As well as the risk of type 2 diabetes from being overweight or obese; and the other health concerns including high blood pressures, cancer and cardiovascular disease; we now know that a BMI of over 40 increases your chance of dying of Covid-19 (should you catch it) by 90%. If your BMI is between 35-40 then it increases your chance of dying by 40%. A sobering thought.

2. Your Race

As mentioned earlier, if you are of South Asian origin, you can be more genetically predisposed to type 2 diabetes and up to six times more likely to develop it than people of Western or European origin. You also have a higher risk if you are African American, Alaska Native, American Indian, Asian American, Hispanic/Latino, Native Hawaiian or Pacific Islander. If this is you, it is even more important to follow all the dietary and lifestyle recommendations in this book. The fact that – culturally – you may be more at risk does not make it inevitable. But it does mean that you may need to be stricter with these recommendations than someone with a lower risk.

Sometimes a genetic predisposition may be helpful in one environment but might not be so helpful when the environment changes. The Pima Indians, for instance, have a genetic makeup that allows them to survive longer than most of us without food. This is known as the 'thrifty genotype'. This 'thrifty gene' (called apolipoprotein E4 (APOE4)) was extremely beneficial in a time when food supply was uncertain. It allows for more cholesterol to be absorbed from food, in order to make the most of every calorie consumed, which is a survival mechanism when food is in short supply.

But, these days, when food is plentiful and abundant, this same gene gives the Pima Indians a distinct disadvantage, rendering them more susceptible to becoming obese and type 2 diabetic as this gene increases the risk of being insulin resistant.[11]

3. Your Age

Your risk of developing type 2 diabetes increases as you get older, but your racial background plays a part here too, with your risk increasing over the age of 25 if you're African-Caribbean, Black African or South Asian, but over the age of 40 if you're white!

Recently updated national guidelines from the US Preventive Services Task Force have suggested that all overweight and obese Americans should be screened for diabetes at 35 years old. The previous guidelines, published in 2015, was to screen at 40 – but the age has been lowered because of the rising rates of type 2 diabetes.[12]

4. Your Gender

Where gender is concerned there's unfortunately bad news whichever sex you are! While men are more likely to develop type 2 diabetes, women can have more serious complications from the condition and a greater risk of death.

Interestingly, it is known that a lower testosterone level in men increases their risk,[13] but the opposite is true in women. This is such an opposite effect and yet the research is unclear about the mechanism causing it.

Women do produce testosterone but usually at very low levels; but those who have a higher testosterone level (as with PCOS) store more fat around their middle and, therefore, also have a higher risk of type 2 diabetes. But, paradoxically, in men, the lower level of testosterone causes more fat to be deposited around the middle (visceral fat) and a greater chance of being insulin resistant – because testosterone helps the body take up more blood sugar in response to insulin. Also, fat cells change testosterone into oestrogen, so the higher your fat percentage as a man the lower your testosterone levels will fall.

Being obese also reduces a protein produced by your liver called Sex Hormone Binding Globulin (SHBG) which, as the name suggests, binds hormones including testosterone and oestrogen in your blood.

Being obese also reduces a protein produced by your liver called Sex Hormone Binding Globulin (SHBG) which, as the name suggests, binds hormones including testosterone and oestrogen in your blood. SHBG controls how much of those hormones are delivered to your body's tissues.

Having low SHBG from a blood test has been shown to predict diabetes[14] and that low SHBG may cause insulin resistance.

5. Your Family History

You're two to six times more likely to get type 2 diabetes if you have a parent, brother, sister or child with diabetes. This does not mean that you will get type 2 diabetes, but your risk is higher.

It is known that family history is one of the strongest risk factors for diseases such as type 2 diabetes[15] and also heart disease and cancer. Of course, you do inherit your genes from your parents (see Your Genetics below) but you also inherit many cultural experiences too and certain patterns of eating (healthy or unhealthy) and lifestyle (e.g. exercise). Your family history is thought to be a good predictor of your risk of type 2 diabetes because your family members represent that unique combination of genetics and environmental factors, the nature and nurture aspects.

You could easily feel fatalistic because you have a strong family history of type 2 diabetes, but research shows that you have so much to gain by putting in the diet and lifestyle recommendations in this book.[16]

6. Your Genetics

It is thought that there could be several genetic mutations that could increase a person's risk of type 2 diabetes:[17]

- If either your mother of father has diabetes your risk increases by 15%

- If both your mother and father have diabetes your risk increases by 75%

- If your non-identical twin has diabetes your risk increases by 10%

- If your identical twin has diabetes your risk increases by 90%

But not everyone who has one of these mutations will get diabetes – because there are always combinations of genetics and environmental factors.

Genetic disorders are often divided into Mendelian and multifactorial traits. In classical Mendelian inheritance, the colour of your hair is dependent on which gene you inherit from your parents and whether that gene is recessive or dominant.

But in multifactorial diseases like type 2 diabetes (and also heart disease, certain cancers and osteoporosis) there can be many contributory factors and whether a gene, or mutation of it, is "expressed" or not (and whether you end up getting the disease) depends largely on your environment and way of life.

It might be easy to think of your genetic make-up being in the hands of fate and then feeling "oh well, if it is all pre-determined there's nothing I can do". But this is far from true.

It is nearly always the case that subtle differences in our personal characteristics are caused by a combination of:

(1) genetic make-up (your genotype), and

(2) the environment in which you live and develop.

A good example of this is a person who inherits the gene for being tall (thanks to their genotype) but fails to reach their true height because of malnutrition (due to environmental factors that intervened). In this way, the environment can affect the intended working, or "expression" as it is called, of that gene. Your individual identifying traits or characteristics (such as your height) are known as your "phenotype" and this is usually the combination of both genetic and environmental influences.

So, it is not true to say we are 'stuck' with all our genes. Research is showing that we are all truly a mix of our genetic make-up and the environment to which our genes are exposed.

Geneticists refer to the 'environment' as everything that is not the genotype (genetic make-up) and so this can include:

• Diet

• Lifestyle

• Culture

• Drugs

• Chemical exposure

• Infections

Basically this 'environment' is anything in your surroundings. Your genes are influenced by your 'environment' and it is this interaction that can make an enormous difference in terms of your health.

The idea of individuals having different responses to the same disease is evident in everyday life. Before the concept of *genotype* and *phenotype* we would have talked about somebody's *constitution*. The person who drank and smoked into their nineties would be praised for having a *strong constitution* and the one who drank and smoked the same amount but died at 45, a weak one. Yet we always realised the significance of the way we lived – whether we smoked or drank a lot – could make that constitution stronger or weaker. It's a cruel fact of life that some people can get away with much more than others simply because of the cards they were dealt at birth.

What this means is that we each have a unique set of genes that might make us more susceptible to certain diseases like type 2 diabetes – but only more susceptible. Even if you have now worked out that you are someone who is more susceptible, by making changes to your diet and lifestyle – changing your environment – you will reduce your risk. In fact, nowhere is the gene-environment interaction more evident than in type 2 diabetes.

There is little doubt that the science of genetics answers that age old question: we truly are a combination of nature AND nurture.

7. Polycystic Ovary Syndrome (PCOS)

PCOS is a hormonal imbalance that affects five to 10% of women of reproductive age across the world, and results in irregular or absent periods, acne, excess body hair, weight gain and problems with fertility. Most women with PCOS have insulin resistance and excess insulin can stimulate the ovaries to produce more testosterone, giving male hormone symptoms.

Unfortunately, statistics show that the risk of type 2 diabetes is four times higher in women with PCOS and that the disease can develop at a much younger age than women without PCOS.[18] Other information suggests the risk could even be seven times higher.[19] And the first line of treatment for women with PCOS is usually metformin (see page 49) an insulin sensitiser which is often the first drug prescribed for type 2 diabetes.

Chapter 4

Getting a diagnosis

"*Knowledge is power. It helps you take control.*"

For many years, a blood test looking at fasting glucose has been the main way of diagnosing type 2 diabetes, meaning that your blood is taken when you have not eaten or drunk anything except plain water for eight to 10 hours. Having eaten before the test will cause glucose to rise and distort the result, and a fasting test shows what your glucose levels are like without food triggering any spike.

The fasting test can be followed up by an oral glucose tolerance test, if there is any doubt over the diagnosis. Again, this means having to fast overnight, before taking a drink containing glucose in the morning. A blood sample is then taken two hours later. In a non-diabetic person, the level of glucose will not be too high. But a high level over 11.1mmol/L indicates diabetes.

These fasting tests used to be the norm and, once diagnosed with diabetes, a test called HbA1c (glycosylated haemoglobin) would be performed every few months – to give an indication of the average blood glucose over the previous two to three months. However, it has now been recommended that the HbA1c test be used instead of fasting glucose to diagnose diabetes, as it seems to be more accurate at identifying those at risk.

You do not need to fast before having a HbA1c test, which means you don't need to worry about the time of day that you are tested. An HbA1c level of 48mmol/mol (6.5%) or more is considered a diagnosis of diabetes.

The HbA1c test detects how much glucose is attached to part of the red blood cells (the haemoglobin) by measuring the amount of glycation (excess glucose) that has affected the haemoglobin.

The problem with glycation is that it causes free radical damage which is linked to premature ageing, heart disease and cancer.

As we have already seen, there is a step before full-blown diabetes known as prediabetes or borderline diabetes. If you have prediabetes and don't take action in changing your lifestyle then, unfortunately, it will progress to become type 2 diabetes. A diagnosis of prediabetes is made when the HbA1c level is 42-47mmol/mol (6-6.4%).

I remember a lovely lady coming to see me in the clinic. She was upset because she'd been given a diagnosis of prediabetes and told by her doctor: 'come back when you are diabetic'! She had come to me because she didn't want to become diabetic and she knew that she was at a stage where her health could go one of two ways. Either it would progress to type 2 diabetes and she would be on medication for life, or else she could reverse the prognosis by changing her diet and looking at her lifestyle. She was very keen to reverse it. How many people just accept that full-blown diabetes is inevitable? Let's be clear: it's not.

It's worth knowing that this measurement of HbA1c has much larger implications beyond indicating your risk of diabetes. It is well known that people with diabetes are more at risk than non-diabetics of developing certain cancers including womb, liver, pancreatic, kidney, oesophageal, bowel, breast and bladder cancer[20] – and new research has looked at whether the level of HbA1c can be used as a predictor for cancer development, independent of diabetes.[21] One study concluded that 'the incidence of cancer (in the diabetic and non-diabetic populations) could potentially be reduced by decreasing glucose levels. This could be achieved by means of appropriate lifestyle or therapeutic interventions, and by imposing stricter recommendations for glycaemic control.

If you would like to find out your level of HbA1c then do get in touch as it can be organised at one of my clinics, see Chapter 26 on Testing.

Testing For Insulin Resistance

There is a more comprehensive blood test which not only measures HbA1c but also other factors that are important to test in relation to type 2 diabetes. This blood test, which is performed on a simple dried blood sample, which is collected at home and then sent to the lab, measures:

- HbA1c – your average blood sugar (glucose) levels for the last three months.

- Insulin – importantly, whether your level is too high – often a sign of insulin resistance.

- Cholesterol – broken down into HDL ('good'), LDL ('bad') and VLDL, very low-density lipoprotein ('very bad'). Eighty per cent of your cholesterol is produced by your liver (only 20% comes from your diet), but the interesting thing about cholesterol is that it can't travel around your body on its own. In order to get to your cells, it is carried in your blood by combining with a protein, called a lipoprotein (lipo stands for fat). It is the LDL (low density lipoprotein, often called 'bad' cholesterol) that carries the cholesterol to your cells and then it is removed and taken back to the liver by HDL (high density lipoprotein, 'good' cholesterol).

If you have too much LDL and not enough HDL, the cholesterol can be deposited on inflamed artery walls – and this causes the furring of the arteries (atherosclerosis) that can lead to blocked arteries. That is why it is important to check not only total cholesterol but also the levels of HDL and LDL.

VLDL is produced by your liver and supplies your body tissues with triglycerides. High levels of VLDL cholesterol have been associated with the development of plaque in the arteries, which restricts blood flow and can increase your risk of stroke or heart disease.[22]

- Triglycerides are created, and stored, in fat cells, from the excess calories that you've consumed but are unable to use as energy.

They are the major form of fat stored in your body, and a source of energy that your body can release when it needs it. It is your VLDL cholesterol that carries the triglycerides to your tissues. But high levels of triglycerides (because you've been unable to use them for energy) are associated with both metabolic syndrome and non-alcoholic fatty liver disease (page 47).

• High-Sensitivity C Reactive Protein, or CRP, is a marker of inflammation that's produced by your liver. A high sensitivity CRP test, as the name implies, is more sensitive than just a standard C Reactive Protein test. The level of CRP increases when there is inflammation in your body and the level can be used to assess your risk of coronary artery disease. But this measurement is also very important for type 2 diabetes, as it has been shown that higher levels of CRP are significantly associated with an increased risk of the disease.

This test is a fasting blood test, which means that you take the blood first thing in the morning without eating or drinking (except water). A kit will be sent to you and you take a finger prick sample of blood at home and then send the sample to the lab for analysis.

For more information on this test see Chapter 26 on Testing.

Chapter 5

Complications

"Diabetes affects your whole body and leads you down a path to serious health consequences."

The aim of this book is to keep type 2 diabetes at bay. I want to help you lower your risk or stop yourself progressing from prediabetes to type 2 diabetes. And if you've already been diagnosed with type 2 diabetes – whether you are on medication or not – I hope to help you manage or even reverse the condition (and it is even possible to come off drugs for diabetes if you make the right lifestyle changes). This is so important, because there are dire consequences to your health if type 2 diabetes is left to progress or worsen. I cannot stress enough how it affects your whole body and leads you down a path to serious health consequences.

These consequences include:

- Vision loss and blindness
- Kidney problems
- Heart disease and stroke
- Loss of feeling and pain (nerve damage - neuropathy)
- Foot problems (sores and infections)
- Skin issues
- Gum problems
- Erection issues
- Non-alcoholic fatty liver disease

Vision Loss And Blindness

Diabetes is the leading cause of new cases of blindness among adults in the US,[23] and results from high blood sugar levels damaging the tiny blood vessels that supply the retina at the back of the eye. Your retina needs a good supply of blood but, if these tiny blood vessels are damaged, it can't do its job of converting light into the electrical signals that your brain converts into images. You are at risk of diabetic retinopathy generally if you have type 2 diabetes, but this risk increases if you also have high blood pressure and/or high cholesterol. Make sure you get your eyes checked every year, and contact your doctor if you are getting blurred vision or floaters (shapes floating in your eyes).

Kidney Problems

Recent research has shown that diabetes is also the leading cause of kidney failure (diabetic nephropathy) in the US.[24] The job of your kidneys is to clean your blood by removing waste products and extra fluid from your body. If this delicate filtering system gets damaged, then the kidney disease can progress to kidney failure and this is life-threatening and requires dialysis or a kidney transplant. It is important to watch out for symptoms such as higher blood pressure, swelling in your feet or ankles, needing to urinate more, persistent itching, nausea and vomiting, and loss of appetite.

If you have diabetes, then make sure your doctor checks you yearly. A simple urine test can detect protein in the urine (proteinuria) which can be the first sign that your kidneys are not working properly and the protein is leaking through the kidney filters and into your urine. A blood test can then check the glomerular filtration rate to see how well your kidneys are functioning.

Heart Disease And Stroke

By damaging your blood vessels, diabetes also enhances your risk of a heart attack or stroke – so do think about other risk factors, too, and make sure you get your cholesterol and blood pressure checked regularly (see Chapter 26).

Peripheral Neuropathy (Nerve Damage)

Nerve damage can manifest as pain, burning, numbness and tingling. This is often first felt in your feet (see below) but can also occur in your hands, legs and arms. Having chronically high blood sugar damages the small blood vessels that supply your nerves and, over time, they too become damaged. These nerves should be carrying messages from your brain to other parts of your body, but they can't. The symptoms can be worse at night, and you might also experience cramps as well as muscle weakness, if the nerve damage is interfering with the usual signals that tell your muscles to move. You could have difficulty walking, getting up from a chair or carrying things. You may even feel unbalanced or unsteady.

Foot Problems

If you have diabetes, please check your feet regularly because your impaired blood supply could lead to numbness and mean that you miss signs of a sore or cut which could become infected and gangrenous. The NHS estimates that 175 amputations resulting from diabetes are performed every WEEK in England. This means that people with diabetes are about 23 times more likely to have a leg, foot or toe amputated compared to those without diabetes.

If you lose feeling in a foot you could even break or dislocate a bone and not realise it! This can alter the shape of your foot and is known as Charcot foot – and, once your foot changes shape, it cannot return to normal.

Skin Issues

Both prediabetes and full-blown type 2 diabetes can cause darkened skin on certain areas of your body – a condition known as acanthosis nigricans. This darkened skin is often found between your elbow and shoulder and, at first, you might think your skin is just dirty or it can feel like velvet. It can also be found on the back of your neck, groin or armpit. You can also develop skin tags (acrochordons), floppy bits of skin that can grow anywhere but are most commonly found on the neck, underarms and eyelids. Skin tags don't necessarily indicate prediabetes, but they can show that your blood sugar is not as balanced as it should be. You might also see patches on your skin that seem like small, raised pimples at first and then turn into patches of hard, swollen skin which can be yellow, red or brown in colour. These are medically known as necrobiosis lipoidica.

You may also have problems with wounds and open sores that are slow to heal (because of the problems with nerve damage and poor circulation caused by the diabetes). Skin infections are common with diabetes, as are 'shin spots' – brown spots, or sometimes lines, most commonly seen on the shins (diabetic dermopathy).

Gum Problems

Having diabetes can also affect your gums and can cause periodontal disease. According to Diabetes UK, you are three times more likely to develop a dental problem than someone without diabetes. This is because excess sugar in your saliva, caused by high blood sugar, enables bacteria to breed and they produce an acid which can not only damage your gums but also attack your tooth enamel.

You can also experience gingivitis (gum inflammation) and a dry mouth (xerostomia) as well as oral thrush.

Oral hygiene is important for other aspects of your health too. It is known that oral health is linked to heart health, and research has shown that those with gum disease are more likely to have narrowing of the arteries. It is thought that the same mechanism could be happening in the brain – and research has shown that people with poor oral hygiene and bleeding gums are more likely to suffer with memory problems.[25] The thinking is that the bugs that cause gum disease enter the bloodstream, setting up an immune system reaction which then produces inflammation and narrows the blood vessel in the heart and the brain.

Make sure you have regular check-ups not only with the dentist but also the hygienist and get into a regular habit of flossing as well as brushing.

Erection Issues

Again, because of the issues with blood vessels and nerve damage, type 2 diabetes may cause sexual problems. It can make an erection difficult because of changes with blood flow and there can also be loss of sensation. Diabetes UK says that men with diabetes are three times more likely to have trouble getting or keeping an erection.

It is easy to see how changes in your blood vessels can impact on so many different systems in your body.

Non-alcoholic Fatty Liver Disease (NAFLD)

NAFLD occurs when fat builds up in the liver, and this is common in type 2 diabetes (about 70%[26]) and anyone who is overweight or obese. Fatty liver can occur when people drink too much alcohol, but this is not the case with NAFLD. NAFLD can increase the risk of heart attacks and stroke and, as type 2 diabetes also increase these risks, this is a particularly dangerous combination to have.

NAFLD progresses through four stages:

1.   Simple fatty liver (steatosis) – fat starts to build up in the liver.
2.   Nonalcohol steatohepatitis (NASH) – the liver becomes inflamed and you might experience pain on the right side of your abdomen.
3.   Fibrosis – fibrous scar tissue forms in the liver.
4.   Cirrhosis – where healthy liver tissue is replaced by the fibrous scar tissue and the function of the liver is affected and causes life-threatening liver failure.

Your liver should contain very little fat, but the diagnosis is NAFLD when fat makes up more than five to 10% of the liver's weight.

The problem is not due to the fats in your diet as you might think – because these are transported into your lymphatic system before they enter your bloodstream.

But, when you have too much sugar and refined carbohydrates in your diet, and your body has so much more glucose (sugar) than it needs for energy (and can't store any more as glycogen), the excess goes to your liver where it is turned into triglycerides (fat).

The other major risk factor for fatty liver is the consumption of high fructose corn syrup/fructose as a sweetener (see page 78). Insulin is not needed to metabolise fructose and it goes straight to your liver which turns it into fat. Fructose triggers lipogenesis (the production of fats, e.g. triglycerides) in the liver which can lead to NAFLD.[27]

NAFLD is usually picked up on an ultrasound scan and you might be recommended to have this done if, from a blood test, your liver enzymes are in the abnormal range. Higher levels of triglycerides in a blood test can also be an indication of a fatty liver and high level of triglycerides can also increase your risk of heart attack and stroke. But NAFLD can present with no symptoms at all. So, it is important to ask to be checked for this if you have type 2 diabetes or are overweight or obese.

The Bottom Line

In order to avoid any of the complications of type 2 diabetes, I cannot stress how important it is to put into place the recommendations, both dietary and lifestyle, from this book.

Chapter 6

Medical interventions

"Few medicines are side-effect free, and it's always better to head off your medical condition through a healthier lifestyle if you can."

I want to say something about the drugs you may be taking – or are due to be taking – for your diabetes. Because, although they may seem like a quick fix to your problem, few medicines are side-effect free, and it's always better to head off your medical condition through a healthier lifestyle if you can. The dietary recommendations and other natural solutions outlined in this book should help you reach this goal – so do let your doctor know what you are doing, so they can help to monitor your progress.

And, if you've been told that you are soon going to need to go on medication if nothing changes, it really is crucial that you take every step you can to avoid going down that route. You will then be in a better position to reverse your disease too.

I am going to cover the different medications for diabetes but, of course, your doctor will suggest the most appropriate one for you. This is just an overview.

Oral Medications

• Metformin

The most commonly prescribed medication for type 2 diabetes is metformin and this will often be the first medication suggested. Brand names for metformin (also known as biguanide) include Glucophage, Metabet, Bolamyn, Diagemet, Glucient and a liquid form of metformin called Riomet.

This is an insulin sensitising drug which works by re-sensitising the body to insulin, reducing the absorption of glucose in the digestive system, and lowering the liver's production of glucose.

But, the USA's Diabetes Prevention Programme found that lifestyle interventions (diet and exercise) were actually more effective than metformin in preventing or delaying diabetes.[28] And the researchers pointed out that, as well as preventing diabetes, these had a beneficial effect on weight, blood pressure and lipid levels (increasing HDL ('good' cholesterol) and lowering triglycerides). Metformin can have a beneficial effect on weight but it does not seem to have any effect on blood pressure or lipid levels.

It is interesting to note that nearly half of adults prescribed metformin stop taking it within a year of being diagnosed with type 2 diabetes, even though they may have HbA1c levels above 7.5%. The biggest fall off was during the first 30 days and no other medication was given instead.[29]

The drop off might be due to gastrointestinal side effects such as upset stomach, diarrhoea and nausea – all of which are common. Metformin can also cause a loss of appetite and a metallic taste in the mouth.

It is worth knowing that if you do take metformin, it increases your risk of having a vitamin B12 deficiency[30] which, in turn, can cause fatigue, diarrhoea, poor memory, pins and needles, menstrual problems, depression and nerve damage.[31]

If you have been on metformin for longer than six months, then I would suggest you see your GP for a blood test to check your level of vitamin B12.

Metformin comes in two types – standard release and slow release. The standard release tablets release metformin quickly into your body so they need to be taken a number of times during the day, whereas the slow release tablets usually only require one tablet with the evening meal.

Metformin does not, on its own, cause low blood sugar

(hypoglycaemia, also known as 'hypos') but it can cause that if it's combined with other diabetes medication.

Some people can have a serious allergic reaction (anaphylaxis) to metformin, so it is important to look out for symptoms such as skin rash, wheezing, swelling of the tongue and lips and trouble breathing. If metformin is not working for you then your doctor will usually prescribe another medication. There are now many medications on the market for type 2 diabetes. The following, taken from information from Diabetes UK, are just a few of the options your doctor may consider for you.

- **Sulphonylureas**

This medication works in a different way to metformin in that it stimulates the cells in your pancreas to make more insulin.

- **Alpha Glucosidase Inhibitor (Acarbose)**

This drug works by slowing down the absorption of sugar and starchy foods in your intestines to slow down the rise in blood sugar after eating.

- **Prandial Glucose Regulators**

Like sulphonylureas, this helps your pancreas to produce more insulin, but it only lasts for a short amount of time, although it works quicker than sulfonylureas. It is taken 30 minutes after eating.

- **Thiazolidinediones (Glitazones)**

This medication is aiming to improve insulin sensitivity.

- **GLP-1s (Incretin Mimetics)**

This medication increases the level of incretins which help your body produce more insulin when needed. They can also reduce your appetite so that makes them helpful for weight loss. Although usually given by injection (see page 53), which is not that convenient, one GLP-1 – Semaglutide (brand name Rybelsus) – is now available in an oral form.

Recent research has shown that 75% of people who received Semaglutide lost more than 10% of their body weight, with more than 35% of them reducing their body weight by up to 2% – the same as weight loss surgery.

The trial involved nearly 2,000 people and they were either given 2.4mg of Semaglutide or a placebo, once a week. They were also asked to follow a reduced calorie diet and to increase exercise.[32] Side effects include nausea and diarrhoea.

• DPP-4 Inhibitors (Gliptins)

This type of drug blocks the action of DPP-4 which destroys the hormone incretin.

• SGLT2 Inhibitors

This one reduces the amount of sugar (glucose) absorbed by your blood.

Did You Know?

Many medications that are commonly used nowadays were first derived from plants (herbal medicine). Aspirin is based on an extract from willow, originally used for pain relief by the Native Americans. Pharmaceutical companies only use the 'active ingredient' of the plant or herb in a pure form as the basis for the drug. Ancient peoples always used, and continue to use, the whole plant. The advantage of using the whole plant is that the side-effects are absent or minimal. That is the big difference between modern and herbal medicine.

The foxglove plant (*Digitalis purpurea*) was used for heart problems. In modern times, scientists have isolated the main active ingredient of the foxglove (digoxin) and put it into tablet form. However, by doing so, they have created a medication with a real risk of side-effects. By using the whole plant, the active ingredient interacts with all the other constituents of the plant, which naturally contains 'buffer' ingredients that

---

counteract any potential side-effects.

In 1772 a traditional herbal medicine in Europe, called *Galega officialis* (also known as goat's rue), was used to treat the symptoms of diabetes. This herb was found to be rich in an active ingredient called guanidine which helped to lower blood sugar. Metformin is a guanidine derivative and has been used to treat diabetes since the 1950s.[33] But metformin comes with side effects, including gastrointestinal symptoms of nausea, diarrhoea, stomach aches and loss of appetite, plus vitamin B12 deficiency.

Injectable Medications

• Exenatide (Bydureon)

This is a once-weekly injection and it works by helping the body produce more insulin when needed. It also reduces the amount of glucose produced by your liver, as well as reducing the rate at which glucose is released into your bloodstream.

Others similar to this are liraglutide and lixisenatide (once daily injections) and dulaglutide (once weekly injection). Semaglutide (brand name Ozempic) is also a once weekly injection, though it is also now available in oral form as mentioned on page 51.

• Insulin

Insulin is normally only used for type 2 diabetes when other medications are not working. It is taken by injection with an insulin pen. Insulin pumps are available, but these are usually only for people with type 1 diabetes. There are different types of insulin, including rapid-acting, short-acting, mixed, intermediate-acting and long-acting. If you need insulin, your doctor will decide the best type for you.

Bariatric Surgery

I hope you may manage to avoid using drugs for your diabetes by following the dietary and lifestyle recommendations in this book

– or that you are at least on the lowest possible dose. But there is another – more drastic – medical treatment for type 2 diabetes and that is bariatric surgery. As well as type 2 diabetes it is also offered to people who need to lose weight and have a BMI of 35 or more.

It works by reducing or bypassing the stomach so that you feel fuller more quickly than usual and so eat less. The surgery also helps with improving insulin sensitivity, reducing absorption of calories, and altering the secretion of the digestive hormones that influence insulin production. This surgery has been shown to be very successful – with blood sugar levels dropping to normal soon after surgery and with people also stopping their diabetes medications quite soon afterwards.

Of course, any surgery comes with risks. So, I would suggest trying the dietary and lifestyle recommendations in this book before embarking on this approach. Immediately after surgery, you would be put on a liquid diet before gradually moving onto more solid food. But, because of the changes in your digestive system, you would be advised to take vitamin and mineral supplements for the rest of your life and nutrient deficiencies are usually monitored every six months.

There are different types of bariatric surgery, and some are more successful for type 2 diabetes than others. The intestinal bypass (also called Roux-en-Y gastric bypass) where the digestive system is re-routed to bypass most of the stomach appears to be the most successful, with diabetes going into remission within days – even before the person has lost much weight. More people who have the intestinal bypass surgery experience remission of type 2 diabetes (82 to 99%) than those who have the gastric restrictive procedures (where either a band is placed around the upper part of the stomach to reduce the volume), or sleeve gastrectomy (where a large part of the stomach is removed).[34] The gastric band procedure is the only one of these that can be reversed later on as the band is inflatable and can be adjusted or removed.

Medications That Increase Your Risk Of Diabetes

Of course, there may be certain medications that you need to take – but make sure you read up on the side effects, because some medications can actually increase your risk of type 2 diabetes, and this is not good if you have already been diagnosed with prediabetes or are at a higher risk.

This is termed drug-induced diabetes. It might be reversible if you discontinue the medication, though sometimes it can be permanent. These medications include statins, corticosteroids, beta-blockers, antipsychotics and thiazide diuretics.

If you are on any of these medications, then it would be worth speaking to your doctor to see if there is an alternative medication that you could take for the same condition that doesn't increase your risk.

I will cover two of the most common medications that you might be taking.

• Statins

Statins are usually prescribed if you have high cholesterol but, unfortunately, as mentioned previously, they can increase your risk of developing type 2 diabetes by almost 50%.[35] Statins seem to have two negative effects on blood sugar at the same time; they decrease insulin sensitivity by 24% and also reduce the ability of your pancreas to secrete insulin by 12%.

Only 20% of the cholesterol in your bloodstream comes from what you eat; the remaining 80% is produced by your liver – and statins work by blocking the production of the cholesterol from your liver. But the question must always be: why is your liver producing too much cholesterol?

There is a strong connection between your liver and blood sugar balance. It is the message that insulin sends out that causes your liver to produce too much cholesterol in general and too much 'bad' LDL cholesterol in particular.

There has been some interesting research on the whole issue of cholesterol and heart disease. In one study, over 130,000 patients who'd been admitted to hospital with a heart attack were found to have lower levels of cholesterol than normal, not higher.[36] Even when the researchers looked at levels of the supposedly 'bad' LDL cholesterol, the people with the lowest LDL levels had twice the death rate three years later.[37]

The key may lie in having optimum levels of the 'good' HDL cholesterol – and it seems that having too much sugar in your blood 'kills' HDL. There is a substance called methylglyoxal (MG), formed by the sugar in your blood, which alters the structure of HDL and makes it less effective. HDL is 'good' because it removes excess levels of bad cholesterol from your body. Higher levels of MG have been found in people with diabetes.[38]

If you need to continue taking statins, then you should know that they not only reduce your liver's production of cholesterol but also reduce the production of co-enzyme Q10. Co-enzyme Q10 is contained in nearly every cell of your body. It is important for energy production in your cells and is vital for heart and muscle function. Not having enough co-enzyme Q10 makes you age faster and can accelerate DNA damage. Even just two weeks on a statin can cause a significant decrease in co-enzyme Q10 levels.[39] It is important that you take co-enzyme Q10 if you are on a statin and it is included in the Blood Sugar (Glucose) Support supplement mentioned on page 134.

• Corticosteroids

These might be prescribed for autoimmune problems such as rheumatoid arthritis and lupus – but they can raise your blood sugar. It should return to normal once you stop taking the drugs, but only if you've taken them for less than three months. But it might cause permanent type 2 diabetes if you have to take the medication in the long term.

PART 2

THE ROLE OF DIET

Chapter 7

Eat to beat diabetes

"Avoid those foods that cause a high rise in blood sugar and eat in a way that keeps your blood sugar as balanced as possible."

You know from the previous chapters what is happening in your body with prediabetes and type 2 diabetes, and my aim now is to show you how changes to your diet can either prevent you from moving from prediabetes into full blown type 2 diabetes, or actually help to reverse full blown type 2 diabetes if you've already been diagnosed with it. Importantly, these dietary changes will also help to prevent prediabetes or type 2 diabetes if you know that your family history puts you at risk.

But let me start by saying that I am fully aware of how daunting the words 'changes to your diet' can be. The media bombards us with information about what to eat and what to avoid – and a lot of what we read is conflicting and confusing. One week we are told we should eat margarine instead of butter. The next it is butter that is the healthiest option. The arguments about fat versus sugar, and whether red wine is good or bad for our health, also rage on. It's little wonder that so many people give up and decide to just eat whatever they like. But, over the course of this chapter, I hope to settle some of these arguments and give you the confidence to make healthy changes that you can live with.

Remember that – as I've shown in the opening chapters of this book – a diet that raises your blood sugar also creates a greater need for high amounts of insulin to be produced, which, over time, causes insulin resistance. With this in mind, your aim must be to avoid those foods that cause a high rise in blood sugar and eat in a way that keeps your blood sugar as balanced as possible.

Remember, too, that being overweight or obese is the main risk factor for type 2 diabetes – so it is important that your pattern of eating helps you to lose weight if you need to, and in a healthy way.

But before we get started on how to improve your diet for the better, I think it is important to dispel a couple of very common dieting myths: firstly, that counting calories is the way to lose weight; and, secondly, that a low fat diet is the healthiest way to do this. Controversial, yes, but these really are myths. Let me explain…

The Myth Of Calories

In the past, there has been a lot of talk about calories, and how cutting calories is the answer to weight loss; and, with weight being the driver for type 2 diabetes, this would appear to be a very straightforward solution. But I am going to suggest that you don't count calories – and that's because not all calories are equal.

A kilocalorie – usually known as a calorie – is, in scientific terms, simply a unit of heat – it's the energy-producing property of food. When we burn food, energy is released as heat. To measure the amount of calories in a particular food, it is burned in a lab and the released energy is used to heat a known quantity of water. A calorie is equal to the amount of energy needed to raise the temperature of one gram of water by one degree centigrade (1°C).

We talk about 'calories in/calories out, meaning that we consume calories in the form of food and drink, and we burn them through our metabolism and physical activity. For a long time now, the perceived wisdom has been that, if the calories you consume are less than those you use up, then you will lose weight. Conversely, if you eat more calories than you expend, you will put on weight.

It's true that this is certainly part of the story, but it's not quite as simple as it seems. Nowadays we know that the source of the calorie – whether it's from fat, protein or carbohydrate – is also an important factor in this equation.

Research from Stanford University 'provides the first large-scale, population-based evidence for the idea that not all calories are equal from a diabetes risk standpoint' and that sugar has 'a direct, independent link to diabetes'. It has been shown that sugar intake is a predictor of type 2 diabetes – irrespective of whether someone is overweight.[40]

The research showed that, for every 150 calories from sugar consumed above the recommended daily calorie intake, the rate of type 2 diabetes was 11 times higher than when the 150 extra calories came from non-sugar foods or drink. Confirmation again that not all calories are equal – it really does depend on where those calories are coming from.

Carbohydrates and protein both provide four calories per gram (0.4oz) while fat provides nine calories per gram, so it would seem logical that the more fat you eat the more weight you will gain. However, that is not actually the case – although some fats are very bad for you, not all are. Relatively "low calorie" sugar is far more harmful to your health and weight.

For many years now, the low-fat diet has been promoted by many organisations both in the US and UK – not only for type 2 diabetes, but also for heart disease and weight loss. Alongside this message, we've seen carbohydrates forming the base of the recommended Food Pyramid – suggesting that these are the kind of foods that we should be eating more of. The pyramid has now been changed, in America, to a plate called MyPlate – but carbohydrates still make up 30% of the plate, although vegetables now make up 40%. Additionally, these American dietary guidelines are at least now saying that half of the grains should be in the form of wholegrains (unrefined carbohydrates) as we know that refined carbohydrates raise your blood sugar more than any other kinds of food.

The UK also uses a graphic of a plate – called the Eatwell plate – as the government's official dietary advice about which foods we should be eating. These guidelines suggest that starchy food should make up over a third of what we eat and that meals should be based on potatoes, bread and pasta or other starchy carbs.[41] There is the suggestion that we should choose higher fibre wholegrain carbohydrates – but no recommendations for how much of these.

As you continue to read through this book, you will understand why I believe this advice needs an urgent update – especially for anyone who could be at risk of type 2 diabetes.

Now, despite what I have just said about low calorie diets and why I do not recommend counting calories, there has been some research into treating type 2 diabetes with a very low-calorie diet that it is important to mention here. This research used liquid meals to replace all normal meals and the meal replacements amounted to around 820 calories per day.[42] The usual daily recommendation is for men to have 2,500 calories a day and women 2,000 – so you can see this is quite a considerable drop.

The liquid meal replacements were classed as being nutritionally complete because they contained vitamins and minerals and were made up of 61% carbohydrate, 13% fat and 26% protein. The programme required quite a commitment, not only in terms of the participants, but also healthcare providers as it included one-to-one attendance for 35 appointments over the two years of the study. The meal replacements were used for 12 to 20 weeks, followed by the gradual reintroduction of solid foods and 'normal' eating, alongside support for long term maintenance.

It was a small study of 149 participants with more than a third of the volunteers achieving remission from diabetes after two years – but the point was made that sustained remission would be dependent on the participants maintaining their new healthy weight.

This study has been considered ground-breaking, as it was previously thought that there was no "cure" for type 2 diabetes, and these remissions, if sustained, show that, in fact, having type 2 diabetes does not have to remain your fate once you've been diagnosed. But I have a number of concerns with preventing or treating type 2 diabetes with such extreme calorie restriction.

Firstly, it is hard to introduce 'ordinary' food once you have been used to just meal replacements and it was clear from the study design that anybody with an eating disorder was excluded. My concern is that eating in such a restricted way for up to 20 weeks could actually push someone into having an eating disorder. There are clear links between following diets like this and developing an eating disorder, and women are particularly vulnerable. This could result in anorexia if they have concerns about putting weight back on after the diet or start binge eating because the diet has triggered ravenous hunger.

I have seen people in my clinic who have followed a meal replacement diet like this for weight loss and, when the diet has come to an end, a number of them have experienced unpleasant side effects such as substantial hair loss and, in some cases, altered heart rhythms.

Secondly, I know the aim is to reverse type 2 diabetes or prevent it from happening if you are at high risk – but you also need a diet that is nutritious and will promote your general health too. Therefore, the food choices that help with type 2 diabetes should also be those that can help to prevent other illnesses like heart disease and cancer into the future. Unfortunately, the ingredients of the meal replacements are not, to my mind, healthy because they contain a number of artificial sweeteners (see page 81) and other ingredients such as maltodextrin (see page 151) which I would suggest you avoid.

There are also concerns from scientists about restricting calories in such an extreme way that they could pose a risk for your long-term health, through changes to your body composition and physiology,[43] as well as your metabolism. (Trying to keep this type of diet going into the future to maintain remission from type 2 diabetes is very difficult and changes in your metabolism from the extreme weight loss can cause you to gain the weight back again.)

The Myth Of The Low-Fat Diet

The prevailing wisdom for many years has been that it is fat that is fattening and causes weight gain. And that it is fat that increases your risk of heart disease; hence we have all been led into buying low-fat and no-fat foods.

This myth started in 1913, when a Russian researcher called Nikolaj Nikolajewitsch Anitschkow showed that when rabbits were fed a cholesterol-laden diet they developed plaque in the arteries (atherosclerosis). He also said that the amount of cholesterol given to the rabbits was directly proportional to the degree of atherosclerosis formation. The greater amount of cholesterol the rabbits were given, the worse the plaque formation. *But,* and this is an enormous but, rabbits do not normally eat any foods containing cholesterol. Only animal foods contain cholesterol. Rabbits are vegetarians, so their bodies are not designed to deal with cholesterol![44]

So, the myth started that excess cholesterol in the arteries causes plaque – which is due to excess cholesterol in the blood which is, in turn, due to fatty foods containing cholesterol in the diet.

Other studies that followed used carnivorous animals fed in the same cholesterol-laden way as the rabbits, but they failed to show that fatty deposits of plaque built up in the arteries.

However, the theory that fatty food causes heart disease was further perpetuated by an American physiologist called Ancel Keys who, in 1970, reported that there was a higher incidence of heart disease in countries with a higher intake of saturated fats.[45]

Keys looked at data from seven countries to come to this conclusion. However, seven is not a large number of countries to look at and also, more crucially, he omitted a number of European countries such as France. France is important for what is known as the 'French Paradox'. The paradox is that the French have a high intake of fatty foods, but a low rate of heart disease. The French also eat less sugar – in fact, the country ranks third to last in terms of sugar consumption compared to other European countries, at

68.5g per person per day compared to England at 93.2 and the US at 126.4g per day.[46]

It was originally thought that wine, especially red wine, was protecting the French from heart problems, but it now seems that the protection is not from the alcohol in the wine but the actual grapes from which the wine is made. Red grapes contain a substance called resveratrol which has been shown in studies to reduce cholesterol levels.[47] And recent research has confirmed that drinking alcohol-free wine gives all the same protective benefits without any negatives from too much alcohol.[48]

(Do remember: there is sugar in wine and, while red wine has the lowest amount – at 0.9g per 175ml glass – a dry white wine can contain 1.4g of sugar and rosé wine between 35-120g per glass. This is not added sugar, though. It is in the grapes and turned by yeast into ethanol during the fermentation process.)

In 1977, avoiding or reducing fat became government policy in the US with the introduction of the McGovern dietary guidelines. In 1983 the UK followed suit.

Changing people's long-held beliefs that fat is bad is not going to be easy, even in the light of new research. It is like trying to turn around a huge ocean liner: the process is going to be very slow, and some experts will still not want to relinquish their old beliefs.

But research is showing why it's imperative that this belief changes – and it needs to change quickly. The epidemic of obesity and type 2 diabetes around the world will only get worse if the wrong advice continues to be given.

In 2015, a study in the *British Medical Journal, Open Heart*, showed evidence that dietary recommendations to reduce fat to less than a third of total energy intake had been introduced to 220 million people in the US in 1970 and to 56 million in the UK by 1983, without the supporting evidence from randomised controlled trials.[49]

I will go on to cover why you need to eat fat as well as discussing which fats are to be avoided in Chapter 14.

Chapter 8

What's wrong with sugar?

"When it comes to insulin resistance and type 2 diabetes, sugar is not your friend."

Are you someone who can always find room for a pudding and thinks a cup of tea or coffee is incomplete without a biscuit or chocolate to accompany it? You're not alone! We are born with a sweet tooth, so we are naturally drawn to sweet food. Breast milk is very sweet and it is thought that this natural attraction to sweetness has evolutionary advantages too. Firstly, sweetness indicates that a food has more calories and, hence, is energy dense – and energy-rich foods would have been vital for our caveman ancestors' survival. And, secondly, sweet tastes tend to be a good indicator that a food is safe to eat – bitter tasting foods are more likely to be toxic and would naturally have been avoided by our ancestors.

But, when it comes to insulin resistance and type 2 diabetes, sugar is not your friend. It is what causes your blood sugar to spike, and more insulin to be produced. And, as I mentioned in the last chapter, research from Stanford University makes it clear that a high sugar intake is linked to the development of type 2 diabetes. Even when the researchers controlled for all other food types – fibre, meat, fruits, oils and cereals – only sugar (in its many forms) was associated with a risk of type 2 diabetes. And this association was so strong that it was independent of how physically active someone was or their alcohol intake or their weight.[50]

A European study has also shown that having just one sugar-sweetened drink a day increases your risk of type 2 diabetes by 22%.[51]

However, artificially sweetened drinks are no substitute for sugar-sweetened ones – because the risks with these are just the same, and they also increase your risk of type 2 diabetes. Research from France tracking more than 66,000 women over 14 years, found that the risk of developing type 2 diabetes was higher for women who drank either artificially sweetened or sugar-sweetened drinks than those who did not. However, the really interesting part was that the risk was even higher for those who drank the artificially sweetened ones compared to the sugar-sweetened ones. Half a litre of artificially sweetened drinks increased the risk by 15%, but 1.5 litres caused a 59% higher risk.[52] Please do not see this as a reason to think of the sugar-sweetened drinks as the healthier option, however. They are anything but!

Wherever you get your sugar – be it from a bag of sweets or a can of soft drink, that sugar is a refined carbohydrate that has been stripped of fibre and has no nutritional value. It is nothing more than a source of empty calories.

To make matters worse, as sugar is devoid of nutrients, your body has to use other nutrients stored in your system in order to digest it. So, not only are you getting absolutely no vital vitamins and minerals from the sugar, but your body is also losing valuable nutrients just by eating it. Hence sugar causes a double whammy on the nutritional front and can actually create nutritional deficiencies.

Roller Coaster

When your body is on a roller coaster ride of fluctuating blood sugar levels you can experience any number of different symptoms including:

- Irritability
- Aggressive outbursts
- Nervousness, fears and anxiety
- Depression
- Crying spells
- Dizziness

- Confusion, forgetfulness, inability to concentrate
- Fatigue
- Insomnia
- Headaches
- Palpitations
- Muscle cramps
- Excess sweating
- Digestive problems
- Allergies
- Lack of sex drive

Check The Label!

When you're looking for sugar on the label of a processed food, remember that it is a substance with many different guises. Generally, the names for different kinds of sugars end in –ose. So, sucrose, lactose, fructose, glucose, maltose and dextrose are all sugar.

The problem is that sugar is not just found in the obvious sweet foods (for example, cakes, sweets, chocolate) but it is also 'hidden' in unlikely places, including savoury foods such as tomato ketchup, mayonnaise and salad dressing. Even apparently healthy foods like fruit yoghurt may contain up to eight teaspoons of sugar in a single portion pot.

The fact that we are born with a sweet tooth and will be drawn to eat (and buy) more of the foods that we find sweet and tasty, has been a boon for food manufacturers. And, because sugar is now very cheap, you'll find it added to many different foods – sweet and savoury – once you start looking for it. Just check out your larder and fridge and see how many labels contain those sugar-related words ending in '-ose'. Shockingly, a lot of these foods will be marketed for children – some of our children's breakfast cereals contain very high amounts of sugar. They are purposely designed to be tempting to children and will often be endorsed by a popular cartoon character. Some manufacturers have reduced the amount of sugar in cereals, but they are still high. Some say that they now have 30% less sugar so it just shows how high they must have been in the first place. And because they taste good and children will eat them, they can be an easy start to the day for many families.

Remember anything ending in 'ose' (glucose, sucrose, fructose, lactose, maltose) is a form of sugar, as are honey, agave, molasses and syrups like corn and rice syrup, not forgetting glucose-fructose syrup (high fructose corn syrup). The higher up the ingredients list, the more sugar the product contains.

In one popular breakfast cereal aimed at children there is both sugar and glucose syrup, and the amount of sugars are listed as 17g in a 100g serving, which is four teaspoons of sugar to start the day. The World Health Organisation (WHO) wants adults to limit added sugar (including honey) to just six teaspoons a day.

A diet that is high in sugary foods of any type will increase your risk for type 2 diabetes. But there are other concerns around sugar that you also need to know about – because these are extra health issues that you face if you develop type 2 diabetes.

Sugar And Cancer

We know that having too much sugar, or glucose, in your blood can lead to insulin resistance and excessive insulin circulating in your system. And we know that insulin is a 'grower' – it can make skin tags grow on your neck and armpits and, unfortunately, it can also have the same effect on tumours inside your body.

High levels of insulin have been linked to cancers of the bowel, liver, pancreas, ovary and womb.[53]

As far back as the 1950s a scientist called Otto Warburg discovered that cancer cells have a different form of energy metabolism to healthy cells.[54] They show an increase in a process called 'anaerobic glycolysis', meaning that they use glucose (sugar) as their primary fuel. So, if your blood glucose levels are high, there will inevitably be excess glucose on which the cancer cells can 'feed'. There's no doubt about it: sugar is fuel for cancer cells.

Insulin Alert!

Insulin is classed as an anabolic steroid (a 'grower or builder' of cells) and one of the things it does is to encourage cells to mutate. It also stops a process called apoptosis, literally 'cell suicide'. Healthy cells are normally programmed to die when they have fulfilled their function. If apoptosis is not happening, then uncontrolled cell division can take place as it does in cancer.

We know that when digestion occurs too quickly (because of a high sugar meal), glucose enters the bloodstream too rapidly. But the initial stimulating 'high' this gives you will quickly pass, causing your blood sugar level to plummet so low that it will make you feel tired and drained. Your body's response is to crave another stimulating fix of sugar to bring your mood and energy back up. And so it goes on... We call it a blood sugar roller coaster and, as we've seen, one of the effects of this roller coaster is to stimulate the release of the stress hormone cortisol. This is bad news because cortisol reduces the number of natural killer cells (NK cells) which normally act like a searchlight, helping your immune system to seek out and identify cancer cells as well as viruses. Cortisol also encourages new blood vessels to attach to tumours (angiogenesis), thus stimulating the tumours' growth.

Even just having higher blood sugar levels significantly increases your risk of getting and dying of cancer, regardless of whether you are overweight or not. This is according to research on over 500,000 men and women with an average age of 44. The bad news is that the connection with blood sugar and cancer is even stronger for women and for fatal cancers.[55]

In one study involving over 49,000 postmenopausal women, researchers found that women whose diets were high in sugar and white flour convenience foods were 87% more likely to develop breast cancer than those on healthier diets – but the risk was particularly strong for women who had used HRT or who did no physical exercise.[56]

Another study found that having higher levels of insulin can increase your risk of breast cancer threefold. Here 5,450 women were divided into three groups depending on their insulin levels and followed over eight years. The group with the highest levels of insulin had the greatest risk and this was again independent of their weight. Being overweight is well known to increase the risk of breast cancer, but these results showed that blood sugar and insulin are the major risk factors.[57]

Scientists have now been able to use their knowledge about sugar and cancer to identify the disease by tracking how sugar is absorbed in the body, with the equivalent sugar content of half a standard size chocolate bar causing tumours to glow on an MRI scan.[58]

All this means that, when you reduce your sugar intake in order to lower your risk of diabetes, you also reduce your risk of cancer by starving malignant cells of their fuel – something that is important to keep in mind if you have already had cancer and are working on preventing a recurrence. Research has shown that bringing blood sugar under control should be part of cancer therapy, as high sugar intake is associated with poor survival rates after diagnosis of early breast cancer.

A Spoonful Of Sugar

Because malignant cells need much more glucose to feed their growth, scientists from the University of Edinburgh in the UK have invented a 'sugar bomb' containing a drug that detonates and destroys cancer cells in seconds while the tumours are greedily gobbling up the sugar. Healthy cells are not harmed by the drug as it only works against the cancer cells which grow fast and need more 'food' than healthy ones. The scientists behind this new treatment are likening it to a 'trojan horse' drug which is capable of hunting down and killing cancer cells in the body.

Sugar And Ageing

A few years back, scientists from the Leiden University Medical Centre in the Netherlands measured the blood levels of 600 men and women aged between 50 and 70. They then showed photographs of these men and women to independent people and found that those with the highest blood sugar (glucose) levels looked older than those with the lowest levels. In fact, people appeared to look five months older for every 1mm/l increase in blood sugar![59] The scientists had controlled for other factors, such as smoking, yet it remained the fact that the higher the blood sugar the older the person appeared.

One reason for this is that, due to a process called glycation, sugar bonds with proteins like collagen and elastin and makes your skin lose its more youthful looking plumpness.

Glycation involves the formation of highly toxic chemicals called Advanced Glycation End-products (AGEs) – and these become deposited in the dermal matrix of the skin,[60] making both collagen and elastin become rigid, stiff and inflexible, so that wrinkles form. Your skin can become discoloured, with brown spots, often known as 'liver spots'. It also becomes generally more dry, dull and fragile.

Glycation is why people with diabetes can age prematurely and why they also often have artery, kidney and nerve damage – because it is just as damaging inside, where it can't be seen, as on the outside where it is clearly visible in the shape of wrinkles.

Poor joint mobility is common in people suffering from diabetes. And, as well as a reduction in elasticity, AGEs lead to reduced tensile strength (how much load the joint can bear without fracturing) and increased stiffness.[61]

I mentioned in Chapter 4 that nowadays, when you are tested for your blood glucose levels, it is recommended that HbAlc (glycosylated haemoglobin) is measured instead of fasting glucose.

Sugar And Heart Disease

I've already mentioned that sugar's impact on insulin can affect your immune system's ability to seek out and destroy cancer and viruses, but another effect it has on the immune system is to 'reprogramme' the stem cells that produce white blood cells, called macrophages. As a result, these macrophages become inflammatory, increasing your risk of developing atherosclerosis – the formation of plaque in furred-up arteries that can cause the arteries to become narrowed or blocked – which can cause a heart attack.[62]

While the normal process, following a meal, is for insulin to send a signal to your liver telling it not to release fats into your bloodstream, because your body is already busy dealing with fat from the meal, another problem that occurs when too much insulin is being released (because you are insulin resistant) is that your liver ignores that message and goes ahead and releases those stored fats (triglycerides).

These triglycerides (a known risk factor for heart disease) are contained in VLDLs (very low-density lipoproteins) which are usually rendered harmless by enzymes in your blood. But the enzymes at that moment are dealing with the fat from your food so the VDLs can end up forming atherosclerotic plaque on your artery walls.

In 2009, the American Heart Association published a scientific statement in their journal *Circulation* entitled 'Dietary sugar intake and cardiovascular health'[63] in which they expressed concern that sugar and refined carbohydrates can increase triglycerides while also lowering levels of HDL, the so-called 'good' cholesterol which would normally remove cholesterol from the arteries. (Your cholesterol is measured as HDL, which is protective and heathy, and LDL, which is 'bad' and increases your risk of heart disease. If HDL is low, cholesterol could build up in the blood vessels.) They also pointed out that high sugar consumption is associated with an increase in inflammation and oxidative stress, both of which increase the risk of heart problems.

Inflammation is the key factor here because, as cholesterol travels around your arteries, it will only start to form plaque if your blood vessels are inflamed – because inflammation damages the lining of the arteries making it easy for the fatty plaque to stick. Over time, this fatty deposit can break away from the blood vessel and cause either a heart attack or a stroke, depending on whether it blocks the blood supply to your heart or brain.

Just recently, in 2021, research conducted by the US National Salt and Sugar Reduction Initiative and published in the medical journal *Circulation*, said that cutting sugar from a fifth of packaged foods and 40% of drinks could prevent more than two million strokes and heart attacks, and three quarters of a million diabetes cases.[64] And not only would there be a reduction in risks of these diseases but also enormous savings (more than $118 billion) in healthcare costs. They also said these changes could give over six million quality-adjusted life years (QALYs), with one QALY equalling one year of life in perfect health. This means that these reductions in sugar can bring about both quality and quantity of changes for people's health.

Are You Addicted To Sugar?

You may think that you couldn't possibly be addicted to sugar. But one of the problems facing people who need to cut back in order to dodge or reverse prediabetes is that sugar is a highly addictive substance – and, as we've seen, it is in most processed foods.

The American Psychiatric Association has a manual entitled the *Diagnostic and Statistical Manual of Mental Disorders* and it suggests that the following list indicates the type of behaviours that could indicate an addiction. Run through this list and look at your behaviour over the last year when it comes to eating sugar and sugary foods.

- Tolerance
- Withdrawal
- The substance is often taken in larger amounts than intended
- A persistent desire or unsuccessful efforts to cut down substance use
- A great deal of time is spent in activities necessary to obtain the substance

- Important activities are given up or reduced because of substance use

- Substance use is continued despite knowledge of having a persistent or recurrent physical or psychological problem that is likely to have been caused or exacerbated by the substance

Easier to make sense of is The Yale Food Addiction Scale which asks the same questions in a slightly different way.

Answer yes or no to the following seven statements.

1. I eat certain foods even if I am no longer hungry.

2. I feel sluggish or fatigued from overeating.

3. My behaviour with respect to food causes me distress.

4. I have had physical withdrawal symptoms such as agitation and anxiety when I cut down on certain foods (not including coffee and tea).

5. I have spent time dealing with negative feelings from overeating, instead of spending time with family, friends, work or recreation.

6. I am consuming the same types or amounts of food despite significant emotional or physical problems related to my eating.

7. Over time, I have found that I need to eat more and more to get the feeling I want, such as reduced negative emotions or increased pleasure.

If you answered 'yes' (and this happens more than three times a week) to the first five, and simply 'yes' to the other two, you need to take a long look at your eating habits, as it is very likely you do have a problem with sugar – and in the next chapter I will show you how you can start to deal with it.

Chapter 9

Weaning yourself off sugar

"The fact that sugar is a food does not make it less addictive than other substances."

Since sugar plays such a big role in the development of type 2 diabetes, cancer and heart disease, you'll want to look for ways you can cut down. But don't be surprised if you find it a struggle to start with. You won't be the first person to suffer with withdrawal symptoms, such as poor concentration, irritability and tiredness.

Sugar is addictive and the fact that it's a food does not make it less addictive than other substances. We do have a natural tendency towards sweet foods so we are inherently drawn to them. And this is same for most animals.

In a study, rats who were induced to become sugar-bingers showed signs of opiate-like withdrawal (as with heroin and cocaine) – such as shakes and tremors – when their sugar was removed. When sugar was introduced again two weeks later, they consumed 23% more than they had before.[65]

Further research, this time on humans at the Harvard Medical School, found similar results. The researchers gave 12 overweight men one of two milkshakes. One milkshake had a high glycaemic index (GI) and the other low, but both tasted the same and contained the same amount of calories. I will discuss the glycaemic index in detail in Chapter 11 but high GI foods are those that cause a rapid rise and then a slump in blood sugar. The milkshakes were given on different days and four hours after the men had the high GI milkshake they were hungrier than those who had the low GI drink. The researchers also watched what happened in the brain in response to the high GI and low GI milkshakes on an MRI scan.

The results were very interesting because the images after the high GI milkshake showed intense activity of a structure in the brain called the nucleus accumbens, which is associated with pleasure eating, reward and craving. The same 'lighting up' of this area of the brain can be seen after people use cocaine and heroin.

The researchers suggest that this supports the argument that food can be addictive and that we do not just eat for our survival and daily energy needs.[66]

With high GI foods, the more you eat, the more you want. Some of my patients call themselves 'carboholics' because they feel they are addicted to carbohydrates like white flour and sugar just as if they were an alcoholic. They have a fair point.

To make it easier to break your sugar addiction, try weaning yourself step-by-step, over a period of days or weeks. It really depends on your personality. It is a bit like someone giving up smoking, some people would rather just stop; others would gradually reduce. The choice is yours.

1. Start with any savoury foods that contain added sugar and remove these from your diet. This might be as simple as just changing the brand so you keep the same food but the ingredients are healthier. Or you might have to ditch that food if there isn't an alternate or make it yourself. Foods to think about are tomato (spaghetti) sauces, mayonnaise, salad dressings, baked beans and soups.

2. The next step is to stop adding sugar of any type (see chapter 10) to your hot drinks and other foods. Some people will sprinkle sugar on to their cereal in the morning when there is already a lot of sugar already added to it (remember to read those packets!) This is similar to people who sprinkle salt on their food before tasting it, when it might be salty enough. Wean yourself off added sugar, gradually diminishing the amount you use each day over a period of days or maybe weeks.

3. Next, take a look at the sweet foods you are eating on a regular basis that contain added or hidden sugar. You might think that a 'live' fruit yoghurt that is a healthy option – but, as we have seen, it can contain up to eight teaspoons of sugar. Buy natural organic yoghurt and drop in or blend in your own fresh or frozen fruit.

Those cereal bars that seem 'natural' may also be loaded with sugar. Sugar is, technically, natural so the marketing is correct but, nonetheless, it is not good for you. There are usually alternative brands you can buy that will be sugar-free, using naturally sweet ingredients such as dates and dried fruits. Dried fruits are high in natural sugar so you need to be careful about eating them just on their own but if they're combined with nuts and other ingredients, they can give you the sweetness that you might be craving.

Also think of the 80/20 rule. The idea is that, if you are eating well 80% of the time, it's okay to indulge for the remaining 20%. So, the occasional slice of chocolate cake at a party is not a big deal: it is what you are eating and drinking on a daily basis that counts. Trying to live by the 80/20 rule makes a healthy diet much more 'doable'. You won't feel so deprived, and will be less obsessed with what you can and can't eat. Over time you may even find that those occasional treats no longer appeal to you – especially if you notice (as can happen) that they leave you feeling tired and irritable afterwards. As you eat less and less refined sugars and carbohydrates, your body becomes more balanced and can become more sensitive to the small effects that different foods have on you. Your taste buds will also change. One of my patients mentioned that after she had ditched the sugar she was at a party and accepted some cake – something she used to enjoy. But now she actually found it so sweet that she had to stop eating it. She said it was almost like it was 'burning' her tongue. You will be familiar with the feeling of a 'sugar rush' which can cause you to become hyperactive after eating or drinking a lot of sugar in a short space of time. Once you've come off sugar the effect of a sugar rush can be even more powerful and fast-acting and you're likely to respond in this way to much smaller amounts of sugar, because your body is no longer used to dealing with it.

Chapter 10

Sweet enough already?

"Artificial sweeteners can actually cause you to gain weight and will increase your appetite."

A closer look at sources of sweetness – be they natural or artificial – will further help you make healthier choices. As ever, I stand by my belief that knowledge is power. Understanding what is happening biologically should help to motivate you and keep you on track when (for example in times of stress, which I will discuss in detail in Chapter 23) those sugar cravings strike.

High Fructose Corn Syrup (HFCS) / Fructose

HFCS, converted from corn, is a mixture of glucose and fructose but can contain up to 90% fructose. It is very popular in America because (partly due to US government subsidies) it is 30% cheaper to use than regular table sugar (sucrose), and the USA has an abundance of corn with which to make it.

HFCS is produced by first making corn starch from corn and then refining the starch into corn syrup. Enzymes are then added to the syrup to change a percentage of the glucose into fructose. In the UK you may find it labelled as glucose-fructose or fructose-glucose syrup on ingredient lists. You will find it in processed foods, drinks, and even some food supplements – and you can also buy pure fructose as a white powder which can used as a sweetener in your own meal preparations.

It was first thought that fructose could be a useful substitute for sucrose (table sugar) and might be helpful for diabetes because it does not cause the release of insulin.

However, because fructose does not use insulin to remove it

from your bloodstream, it goes straight to your liver which has to metabolise it, in the same way as it does alcohol. So, it can make you gain weight, increase your appetite and also give you fat around the middle. The metabolism of fructose is also twice as fast as glucose metabolism so the toll on your body is harder.

There are other problems with fructose too:

- It interferes with your production of hormones like leptin, which should send you a signal telling you that you have eaten enough. When leptin is suppressed, it means you have far less control over your appetite because you will still feel hungry. Adding insult to injury, fructose can also raise levels of a hunger hormone called ghrelin, increasing your appetite!

- It triggers lipogenesis (the production of fats such as triglycerides) in the liver which can, in turn, lead to the increasing incidence of non-alcoholic fatty liver disease.[67] When severe, this develops into non-alcoholic steatohepatitis which can lead to severe scarring of the liver (cirrhosis) and an increased risk of liver cancer (see page 47).

- It is converted into unhealthy fats such as LDL ('bad') cholesterol and triglycerides. And, as high levels of triglycerides are associated with type 2 diabetes, it's ironic that many people switch to fructose instead of sucrose in an effort to stop their insulin spikes.

So, What About Fructose In Fruit?

Do these issues around fructose mean we should be avoiding fruit? Not at all. HFCS and refined fructose are known as 'unbound' or 'free', but when the fructose is contained within fruit it is bound up with the vitamins and minerals, fibre, fatty acids and other sugars within that food, so it does not have the same effects on the liver as the powdered refined fructose, as it is released more slowly and generally eaten in small quantities.

In fact, recent research has shown that people who consume two servings of fruit a day have a 36% lower risk of developing type 2 diabetes over the next five years than those who consume half a serving. And those who eat more fruit have been shown to have better markers of insulin sensitivity, meaning that their bodies need to produce less insulin in order to lower their blood sugar levels. However, these benefits do not apply to fruit juice. You need to eat the whole fruit.[68] We can digest the amounts of fructose we get from eating fruits but, in larger amounts from fruit juices, the fructose will move to the liver and be turned into fat.

Research comparing the effect of fructose-sweetened drinks with glucose-sweetened drinks on obese people found that those who had the fructose-sweetened drinks with their meals had triglyceride levels 200% higher than those who drank the glucose-sweetened drinks with their food.[69]

We know that glucose-sweetened drinks are not healthy as the glucose (sugar) is going to hit your bloodstream too quickly, so I am definitely not recommending them but it was interesting to see that the fructose-sweetened ones caused such a high rise in triglycerides. You really want to avoid both types of sweetened beverages.

So, what about drinking wine with a meal, you may wonder. Interestingly, it has been shown that among people with well-controlled type 2 diabetes following a Mediterranean diet, red wine drinkers had a modest improvement in HDL ('good' cholesterol) compared to those drinking white wine or mineral water.[70] However, I think it is important to have a break from alcohol initially – especially for the first six weeks or so of starting the dietary changes – to give your body the chance to rebalance itself. And don't be misled by the research: although these study participants saw healthy benefits from drinking wine, it was just one unit (125ml or 5oz) of red wine and, importantly, the participants had been chosen because they already had well-controlled type 2 diabetes, and they were following the Mediterranean diet. Also, as we now know the benefit from the red wine is actually from the antioxidants in the grapes; you could achieve the same benefits from drinking alcohol-free wine.

This option gives you all the protective benefits without any negatives from too much alcohol.[71]

Artificial Sweeteners

You might think, then, that artificial sweeteners would be a better choice than sugar as they have no calories and are not going to cause a rise in blood sugar and an increase in insulin.

But they can actually cause you to gain weight and will increase your appetite.[72] When you eat something sweet it usually comes with a bulk of calories. But artificial sweeteners have no calories, so your body sets off to find calories elsewhere. It does this by increasing your appetite and giving you cravings.

Sugar activates the sweet receptors on your tongue and increases dopamine in your brain – and the artificial sweeteners also have this effect. But sugar has a secondary effect, causing an increase in glucose. Artificial sweeteners have no effect on your blood sugar or may even give you low blood sugar (hypoglycaemia) which leaves you feeling hungry, unsatisfied with what you have eaten, making you eat more the next time.

When rats are fed artificial sweeteners, they take in more calories and weigh more, and – even more worryingly – this weight is made up of increased body fat. The researchers commented: 'These results suggest that consumption of products containing artificial sweeteners may lead to increased body weight and obesity by interfering with fundamental homeostatic, physiological processes.' Basically, the artificial sweeteners change the animals' appetite control and inner sense that they have had enough to eat.[73]

Two groups of rats were fed exactly the same number of calories, but one group was given either saccharin or aspartame (artificial sweeteners) and the other group was given sugar (sucrose). The rats given the artificial sweeteners gained more weight than the rats eating sugar.[74]

In a recent study, people were given a 300ml drink containing just water or one sweetened with sugar or one sweetened with sucralose. Within two hours of finishing the drinks, the participants gave blood samples and had an MRI scan while being shown pictures of burgers, sweets and doughnuts. Then they were offered unlimited access to a buffet.

Women and obese people showed more activity in the brain regions responsible for cravings and appetite after consuming the sucralose drink than the sugar sweetened one. Also, after the sucralose drink, those participants had a decrease in the hormones that tell a person that they felt full. And women ate more at the buffet after the sucralose drink.[75]

We know that people who drink two or more diet drinks a day have waist circumference increases 500% greater than people who don't drink diet drinks.[76]

However, it is not only your waistline you have to worry about with artificial sweeteners. The increased risk of type 2 diabetes is the major problem. Scientists go further and say that these sweeteners have the effect of 'inducing metabolic derangements'.[77] They are altering how your body functions which then puts you at risk of major life-threatening illnesses.

The suggestion is that artificial sweeteners (or non-caloric artificial sweeteners as they are often called) are causing glucose intolerance by altering the beneficial bacteria in the gut.[78] We know that gut bacteria have a role to play in insulin resistance, obesity, non-alcohol fatty liver disease and type 2 diabetes[79] and that there is a difference in the gut bacteria composition in normal and overweight people.[80] We will look at this in more detail in Chapter 18.

The artificial sweeteners can turn your healthy gut bacteria into harmful pathogens (disease causing) and potentially cause serious health problems such as life-threatening sepsis (blood poisoning) and other infections, by crossing your gut wall and getting into your bloodstream. They can also accumulate in your liver, spleen and lymph nodes and cause other infections.

Research has shown that even just two cans of diet soft drinks can significantly increase the ability of these harmful bacteria to invade the wall of the intestine.[81]

There are a number of different artificial sweeteners – aspartame, saccharin, acesulfame-K and sucralose – and I would strongly suggest you avoid them all.

Natural Sweeteners

Of course, you may still want some sweetness added to your food – so what are your best options?

If you are making cakes, think of ways other than sugar to add sweetness. For example, you could add carrots, raisins, dates, figs or bananas as natural sweeteners. Many people now make wonderful cakes from naturally sweet vegetables such as beetroot and carrot. For apple pies or crumbles, use eating apples instead of cooking apples so you do not need to add sugar – and you could always add raisins or sultanas to make a pie or crumble that little bit sweeter.

Some spices like cinnamon and vanilla also add sweetness and flavour, enabling you to reduce the amount of other sweetener in a recipe, or remove it altogether. Another way to reduce the amount of sugar when cooking and baking is to add lemon or orange zest – but make sure to use organic fruit, as pesticides and chemicals can be concentrated in the skin. As your taste buds grow accustomed to doing without the very powerful taste of refined sugar you will come to appreciate the natural sweetness of vegetables and fruits.

With regards to natural sweeteners, I have put stevia first because it can have the same negative effect on your appetite as the artificial sweeteners above.

• Stevia

Stevia is derived from the leaves of a South American plant of the same name. It has been used for centuries as a sweetener in South America and for 40 years in Japan. Stevia is 200 to 300 times sweeter than table sugar (sucrose). It is not absorbed through the digestive tract, is considered to have no calories, and does not raise blood sugar, because it has a glycaemic index of 0 (see Chapter 11), so it appears a good choice for type 2 diabetes.

However, although pure stevia is more natural than artificial sweeteners, it can still prime your body to expect the corresponding number of calories that should normally accompany the level of sweetness. As with artificial sweeteners, when that calorie hit doesn't happen, your body sets off to find those calories elsewhere, increasing your appetite and causing weight gain.

Also, research has suggested that stevia can have a negative effect on the beneficial bacteria in your gut. It doesn't seem to kill the good bacteria, but it can result in an imbalance, because it stops them communicating with each other to regulate your body's functions.[82]

Another word of warning: some products can contain dextrose as well as stevia. If you eat one of these, you will be additionally consuming a refined sugar which will affect your blood sugar level and also increase insulin.

• Agave

This sweetener has become very popular over the last few years. In theory it should be a good natural sweetener as it comes from the agave plant in Mexico, where the sap would have been boiled for hours to obtain the sweet syrup. The problem is that, when something is commercially produced, corners are cut to make a product financially viable.

In order to produce agave on a commercial scale, the agave is made from the starch of the root bulb and the final product is just refined fructose because it is made by the same process that converts corn starch into High Fructose Corn Syrup. It is even said that the fructose content is higher than the high fructose corn syrup (see page 78) – and is actually up to 90% fructose.

• Honey

Although this is a natural sweetener, honey is a simple sugar, primarily made up of glucose and fructose, and so is absorbed into your blood stream quickly, so not good for preventing or treating type 2 diabetes.

Research has looked at the effects of giving honey to patients with type 2 diabetes over eight weeks, compared to a control group.[83] Although the honey helped with reducing cholesterol, it caused a significant increase in HbA1c so can't be recommended for anyone working on preventing or treating prediabetes or type 2 diabetes.

Sadly, honey cannot even be recommended as a natural food – because bees gather their nectar from flowers over summer, and honey is often harvested from the hives in the autumn, but the bees will then struggle without food over the winter. So, they are fed a substitute for nectar – and this is white sugar dissolved in hot water! Some 'natural' beekeepers do leave enough honey in the hive so the bees can feed until the spring – but commercial beekeepers know they can sell the honey for more than the sugar water costs, so they're not going to feed it to the bees over the winter.

All this means that you may not be buying 'pure' honey, even when the label suggests it is pure, because the sugar water gets mixed up with the honey in the hive – so the raw material for the honey is simply white sugar. Unfortunately, it is impossible to tell from the honey label whether the bees have been fed sugar over the winter months.

In America, they have even been using High Fructose Corn Syrup (HFCS) instead of sugar water to feed bees over the winter because it is cheaper – and there are now concerns about how this practice may impact on the bees' health. Hydroxymethylfurfural (HMF) – a heat-formed contaminant found in HFCS – is toxic to bees and can cause ulceration of their digestive tract.[84] It's thought it could be one of the causes of the widespread death of bees.

• Xylitol, Sorbitol And Erythritol

These are all classed as sugar alcohols (polyols) and their main side effect is diarrhoea and bloating, as it ferments in the digestive system and would not be recommended for anyone following the FODMAP diet for IBS.

What Is A FODMAP?

The FODMAP diet stands for **F**ermentable, **O**ligo, **D**i, **M**ono-saccharides **A**nd **P**olyols and it involves restricting certain fermentable foods that cause symptoms for people with IBS (Irritable Bowel Syndrome).

FODMAPS include oligo-saccharides (*galacto-oligosaccharides* and *fructans*) such as lentils, chickpeas, kidney beans, broccoli, and wheat; *disaccharides* (lactose) including milk, yoghurt, soft cheeses; *monosaccharides* (fructose) like apples, pears, honey, fruit juices; and *polyols*, for example sugar alcohols like sorbitol and xylitol.

• Xylitol

Xylitol in particular has gained popularity over the last few years. It is sold as a white powder and is considered natural because it occurs naturally in plants. It is low in calories and does not need insulin to be metabolised in the body.

Xylitol in found in the fibres of many plants including sugar cane, corn cobs and birch, and is made from the hydrogenation of a sugar called xylose which is produced from the fibre of the plant. The word 'hydrogenation' rings warning bells as we have been moving away from hydrogenated fats over the years after we found out about the health risks associated with them. There may be concerns about hydrogenated sugar in years to come.

The whole process of making xylitol is very complex and seems very far away from being 'natural' when the process requires the use of nickel catalysts.

• Sorbitol

Like xylitol, sorbitol is a sugar alcohol (polyol) and is often used in foods designed for diabetics because it is metabolised slowly. It is usually made from corn syrup but also occurs naturally in stone fruits such as prunes, plums and dates. Like some other sugar substitutes, it is a very heavily processed product, and hydrogenation is part of the process.

• Erythritol

Erythritol is also a sugar alcohol like sorbitol but, in small amounts, it is supposed to cause fewer digestive upsets because it is a smaller molecule than sorbitol and 90% of it is absorbed in the small intestine and then passed out through the urine. But there are individual variations with some people still experiencing stomach upsets or diarrhoea even with smallish amounts of erythritol.

All of these sugar alcohols can be used safely for type 2 diabetes. They are heavily processed and, therefore, not as natural a food as I would normally recommend – but they could be a good compromise when you need to use a sweetener. I would suggest using these in moderation and they could be used as a sweetener in cooking. Research has suggested that people can tolerate between 10 and 30g of xylitol a day without it causing digestive problems.[85] The research also stated that using 'xylitol in a beverage (apart from just as a sweetener in tea or coffee) cannot be recommended'. But it is considered OK in foods where there is a good amount of fibre.

• Maple Syrup

Maple syrup is made from the sap of maple trees by making a hole in the tree and collecting the syrup.

It is suggested that it has antioxidant and anti-inflammatory properties. A number of the syrup's antioxidant polyphenols inhibit the enzyme that converts carbohydrates to sugar, which is relevant to type 2 diabetes and weight gain. An antioxidant compound called glucitol-core containing gallotannin (GCG), which is only found in maple syrup, has anti-diabetic potential.[86] And many of the antioxidants found in maple syrup which can help prevent the ageing of our body's cells aren't found in other natural sweeteners.[87] It contains bioactive compounds with health-promoting benefits, not only antioxidants but also substances that are antiproliferative and antimutagenic[88] meaning that, unlike sugar, it won't stimulate cancer growth.

Maple syrup is primarily made up of sucrose with very small

amounts of fructose and glucose.[89] If you are prediabetic I would suggest using it very sparingly, just for sweetening when you need a treat, and always have it with foods containing fat and protein – so, for example, in a cake made with eggs and butter to slow down the release of the sugar – but I would suggest you avoid it for at least six weeks if you are working on reversing type 2 diabetes.[90]

Research has looked into whether maple syrup is a suitable sweetener in the management of type 2 diabetes. The research was performed on rats and showed that maple syrup inhibited the absorption of glucose from the small intestines, and the authors stated 'maple syrup might help in the prevention of type 2 diabetes'.

Also, even if you are using it sparingly make sure it is 'pure maple syrup' and not 'maple-flavoured syrup', which may not contain any maple syrup at all. Ingredients of one of these maple-flavoured syrups that I've seen includes invert sugar syrup, colour (150d) and maple flavouring, while another has water (the first ingredient), caramel colour, alcohol, vanilla extract (vanilla bean extractives in water), alcohol and corn syrup, molasses solids, corn syrup solids, natural and artificial flavour, sugar and sulphiting agents. Compared to pure maple syrup, any of these combinations could spike your blood sugar.

Maple syrup is my sweetener of choice. I use it when I'm baking, and drizzle it over the top of crumbles to give it a lovely, browned effect. The evidence is suggesting that it may have anti-diabetic properties but some of the research has been done on rats and not humans so maybe see how your body reacts to maple syrup by just monitoring your blood sugar level after eating it.

• Malt Syrups

Malt syrups can be made from rice or barley and are traditionally made from sprouted grains. Again, if you are prediabetic I would suggest using them sparingly and only with other foods – but avoid them completely if you are type 2 diabetic.

• ## Yacon Syrup

This is a sweetener made from the sweet root of the yacon which is a member of the sunflower family, also known as the Peruvian ground apple. It tastes like a cross between an apple and a pear. Yacon contains good amounts of vitamins and minerals and also a prebiotic called FOS (fructooligosaccharide) which helps to feed the beneficial bacteria in your digestive system.

It is very low GI because the sweetness comes from the prebiotic FOS, and has been shown to lower blood sugar levels in older people[91] and has helped decrease body weight, waist circumference and insulin in obese and pre-menopausal women.[92]

It is best to check with your doctor before using yacon, but it seems one of the best sweeteners to use with type 2 diabetes. Yacon has also been used to lower the blood sugar response after eating.[93] When given to women with their breakfast, compared to just breakfast on its own, the addition of yacon lowered both glucose and insulin after eating. Yacon can used in baking, and also as a liquid sweetener as a substitute for honey – but it may not be suitable for people with IBS due to its high FOS content.

• ## Palm And Coconut Sugar

Palm sugar – also known as jaggery – is made from the palmyra palm tree. The palm flowers are tapped to release the juice which is then boiled down to produce the syrup, which is then allowed to crystalise.

It is a traditional Ayurvedic ingredient and contains good amounts of B vitamins (including a plant source of B12) and also potassium, zinc, iron, manganese and antioxidants such as polyphenols, flavonoids and anthocyanidins.

Coconut sugar, also known as coconut palm sugar, is produced from the sap of the flower buds of the coconut tree. It is also found in liquid form as a syrup as well as crystals. Coconut syrup is also known as coconut nectar and coconut blossom syrup.

To obtain the sap, the tree is tapped as in the palm sugar and minimally heated in order to allow moisture to evaporate to form the syrup. When the syrup cools down it crystalises.

Like palm sugar, coconut sugar is rich in nutrients such as the B vitamins, magnesium, calcium, potassium, zinc, 17 amino acids, short chain fatty acids, polyphenols and antioxidants, and it has a nearly neutral pH. It also contains inulin which, like FOS, is a prebiotic and helps to feed beneficial bacteria.

Both sound good options – however, as there is not much research on either of their effects on blood sugar, I would be wary of using them if you have type 2 diabetes or monitor your blood sugar level if you want to try them.

• Allulose

This is a fairly new sweetener and occurs naturally in a few foods such as figs but in small amounts. Unlike xylitol, sorbitol and erythritol it is not a sugar alcohol and doesn't cause the digestive discomfort that these can cause. Allulose (also called psicose) is absorbed by the body but not metabolised so is virtually calorie-free and has a low glycemic index. It does not affect blood sugar and also slows down the digestion of other carbohydrates, so lowers the glucose response.

Allulose has been shown to lower both glucose and insulin levels in healthy subjects.[94] But further research needs to be performed on people with type 2 diabetes.

Allulose has been approved by the USA's Food and Drug Administration (FDA) but is not yet available in Europe or the UK as it has to be approved as a Novel Food.

I would suggest, then, that if you have already been diagnosed with type 2 diabetes, you avoid stevia, agave, honey, coconut and palm sugar and malt syrups. You could try maple syrup (checking your blood sugar level), yacon syrup and also erythritol, xylitol, sorbitol – but these three sugar alcohols seem to be more refined than yacon so are not as natural in that sense. If you have prediabetes you could try the other natural sweeteners – but sparingly.

Chapter 11

Understanding Glycaemic Index and Glycaemic Load

"Eating slow-release, unrefined carbohydrates helps to balance your blood sugar."

You'll know by now how damaging sugar – and any other food that causes your blood sugar level to spike – can be for your health, but how sure can you be that you are taking sufficient action to keep your diet within safer sugar parameters?

Well, you could start by looking at where your foods sit on the 'Glycaemic Index'. This is a measure that gauges the speed at which your body metabolises one food compared to another, and was conceived by Dr David Jenkins in 1981 in a paper he wrote for the *American Journal of Clinical Nutrition,* in which he suggested that not all carbohydrates were broken down at the same rate and that those that were broken down more quickly would cause a high rise in blood sugar.[95]

A fast-burn food has a high GI and will raise your blood sugar quickly; a slow-burn food has a low GI. However, if all that seems too technical and time-consuming, you could think simply in terms of whether the carbohydrate you're choosing to eat is refined or unrefined – and choose unrefined every time.

On Dr Jenkins' scale, glucose was given a GI of 100 because it causes the quickest rise in blood sugar, and 50g (2oz) of various carbohydrates were then compared with 50g (2oz) of glucose. According to some of the initial results, ice cream registered as a better food for diabetics than wholewheat bread! However, in 1983, other researchers compared the same carbohydrates and got different results. Some experts believe that the results depend on the person's level of blood sugar at the time of the test. Another flaw is that carbohydrates were being tested in isolation, unlike 'real-life' eating.

By 1988 the standard against which all foods were compared had been changed from sugar to white bread but, in time, doubts began to surface again about the accuracy of the GI. The problem is that a number of factors can affect the reproducibility of a GI measure, including the ripeness of the food; the physical form of the food (mashing a 2.5cm (1in) cube of potato increases its GI by 25%); and variability within food classes (e.g. different shapes of pasta, consistency, cooking, etc).

So, the GI is not very helpful. It tells us how quickly that carbohydrate turns into sugar but it does not say how much carbohydrate a particular quantity of food contains. This explains such bizarre contradictions as chocolate (GI 48) having a lower GI than watermelon (GI 72). A GI of 55 or less is low, while 56 to 69 is medium and 70 or more is high.

Glycaemic Load (GL)

A new measure called the Glycaemic Load (GL) was introduced to overcome some of the problems with GI, and this takes into account how much of the carbohydrate is in the food. The real impact on your blood glucose levels will be determined by both the quality (GI) and the quantity (GL) of the carbohydrate.

People were even avoiding carrots because they had a GI of 48, the same as chocolate. But the GL of carrots is 3.9 compared to 14 for chocolate.

There is a good example of the effect of GL when you're choosing whether to have a portion of white rice or couscous with a meal. One hundred and thirty grams (130g) of cooked white rice will provide 40g of carbohydrate and has a GI of 85. But a typical portion of couscous will be 200g (a bigger portion than the white rice) and this provides 45g of carbohydrate and has a GI of 60.

Doing the maths: To calculate the GL of both the white rice and couscous, multiply the grams of carbohydrate by the food's glycaemic index and then divide that answer by 100.

Hence:

Glycemic load of white rice portion

= GI x carbohydrate / 100

= 85 x 40 / 100

= 34

Glycemic load of couscous portion

= GI x carbohydrate / 100

= 60 x 45 / 100

= 27

The smaller portion of rice has less carbohydrate content than the couscous but the couscous has a lower GL which will cause less of a rise in blood sugar than the white rice even though there is more.[96]

The University of Sydney defines low, medium and high glycaemic loads as follows:

- **Low glycaemic load (low GL):** 0 to 10
- **Medium glycaemic load (med GL):** 11 to 19
- **High glycaemic load (high GL):** 20 and over

Any foods that are high in sugar and refined carbohydrates are going to have a high GL.

How Does The Glycaemic Index/Load Work In Everyday Life?

Eating slow-release unrefined carbohydrates not only helps to balance your blood sugar but also benefits your heart and reduces or prevents diabetes.[97]

Research has shown that obese people who eat even *unlimited* quantities of low GI foods lose more weight than obese people on a low fat, low calorie diet.[98] So yes it does work.

Yet, as fascinating as the GI and GL are, I don't think it is a good idea to swap one set of restrictive numbers for another. Having persuaded you to stop thinking about calories, the last thing I want is for you to start obsessing about GI and GL.

The easiest way to think about it all is this: if the food is refined (stripped of fibre) then it is going to hit your blood stream faster and the higher your blood sugar will rise in response to it. The consequence of this will be that your pancreas will produce more insulin to deal with it and, the bottom line, insulin is your fat storing hormone.

Interestingly, whole grains also contain 'enzyme inhibitors' – substances which delay the digestion of starch and sugar, stop the increase in blood sugar levels and so effectively reduce the glycaemic response. They have a similar action to the drugs given to help control type 2 diabetes (alpha glucosidase inhibiting medications), slowing the release of glucose into the blood through the delayed digestion of carbohydrates.

So, when you eat an unrefined, starchy carbohydrate, do have some protein with it (either animal or vegetable based) as this automatically lowers the GI response, slowing down the rate at which the food gets digested. For example, think about a little hummus, cheese or nut butter on your oatcake, or some nuts and seeds and natural yoghurt on your wholegrain muesli. Drizzling oil on a starchy carbohydrate can also lower the GI, as can adding vinegar or lemon juice (by as much as 20-40%). Vinegar is also thought to slow down the rate at which food leaves your stomach.

Here are some more examples of the GL in different foods. You can lower them by making sure you've always got a protein and/or fat with the carbohydrate.

Glycaemic Table

Food	Glycaemic Index (GI)	Serving size (grams)	Glycaemic Load (GL)
Baguette, white	95	30	15
Bread, white	71	30	10
Bread, wholegrain	51	30	7

Food	Glycaemic Index (GI)	Serving size (grams)	Glycaemic Load (GL)
Porridge (oatmeal)	55	250	13
Cornflakes	93	30	23
Quinoa	53	150	13
Rice, white	89	150	43
Rice, brown	50	150	16
Apple	39	120	6
Orange	40	120	4
Banana	62	120	16
Dates, dried	42	60	18
Grapes	59	120	11
Lentils	29	150	5
Cashew, salted	27	50	3
Peanuts	7	50	0
Spaghetti, white, boiled	58	180	26
Spaghetti, brown, boiled	42	180	17
Hummus	6	30	0
Potato, white, boiled	82	150	21
Sweet potato	70	150	20
Parsnips	52	80	4
Pizza, white dough, parmesan cheese and tomato sauce	80	100	22

So, what – if anything – could you do to mitigate the effect on your blood sugar level if you've slipped up and had a pizza, doughnut or pasta dish? Well, the first thing you need to know is that you'd have to act fairly quickly by snacking on some protein as soon as you can. The issue is more serious with the doughnut and pasta as the pizza will have cheese (protein) on it. In this scenario, a doughnut is your worst choice because it combines white flour with sugar and often even more sugar in the jam. Unfortunately, there's not much you can do to offset that one – except to maybe eat it slowly, chew well, and maybe follow up with some nuts for protein. Pasta is just white flour but you could have some hummus or nuts to offset it. Though, really, I don't want to recommend ways to help you cheat, as these will not help in the long term. These blood sugar 'solutions' all carry risks of their own, by pushing up your calorie load and encouraging weight gain. So, you can see how it really is better to just avoid these very highly processed foods.

Chapter 12

The question of carbs

"Reduce or eliminate your refined carbohydrates and include more whole versions, for example brown rice instead of white."

So, you've stripped your larder of foods containing sugar and you now know that refined carbohydrates – white bread, pasta, biscuits, cakes, pizza, pies, breakfast cereals and white rice – are high on the GL scale. This is the next group of foods you need to tackle.

These are foods that have been processed so that the fibre has been removed – along with many of the nutrients that they may have originally contained.

Normally, carbohydrates should provide you with energy. But when they have been refined, they cause your blood sugar to spike quickly – because there is nothing to slow them down.

If you switch from these quick-release white carbohydrates to slow-release whole food alternatives (wholemeal bread, oats, brown rice, etc.), you will create a steady, gradual rise in your blood sugar. Your body, and more importantly your pancreas, hardly has to respond at all – having to release only a small amount of insulin to deal with it.

And, if you need more convincing that this is a worthwhile dietary tweak, consider the findings of a study in the *British Medical Journal* that spanned 16 years and looked at diets from 21 countries around the world, with over 130,000 participants.

For the purposes of this study, grains were classed in three groups: refined grains (pasta, noodles, white bread, cereals, baked goods, etc.), whole grains (whole grain flours like buckwheat) or cracked whole grains (steel cut oats) and white rice.

The results of the study were sobering: eating over seven servings of refined grains a day was associated with a 27% increased risk of early death, a 33% greater risk of heart disease and a 47% greater risk for stroke.[99] White rice was significantly associated with a higher risk of type 2 diabetes.

A recent study also showed that including wholegrains in your diet slows down so-called middle age spread by a half. This research, from Tufts University in Boston, studied more than 3,000 people for 18 years. And it wasn't just the benefits on waist size from eating unrefined carbohydrates. Blood sugar levels also benefitted greatly – as fasting blood sugar level was three and a half times higher in those with a low intake of wholegrains.[100]

Why Fibre Is So Important

It was originally thought that the only role of dietary fibre was to speed up the passage of food residues through the intestines and, hence, prevent constipation. But it has many other benefits too.

- Fibre binds to water and increases the bulk of your stools, so that they are easier to eliminate from your body. It also prevents putrefaction of food which can result if food stays in your bowel too long. Putrefying food will ferment, causing a build-up of gas, leading to problems like bloating and flatulence.

- It also increases your feeling of fullness and removes toxins from your body. By filling you up it helps you to feel more satisfied with what you have eaten and lessens the tendency to overeat.

- Fibre also determines how much oestrogen is stored and how much is excreted – soluble fibre binds to oestrogen so that it is excreted efficiently. As such, chronic constipation has been linked to breast cancer as it has been shown that regular bowel motions are associated with more excretion of oestrogen and lower levels in the blood.[101] Toxic waste products that are not eliminated properly can end up stored in your body's fatty tissue, including the breasts.

- It also increases the amount of time you spend chewing food, hence slowing down eating. The first part of digestion starts in your mouth so chew well and your food will be digested better. (Also, your brain takes 20 minutes to register that you are full so by eating more slowly you will consume less food and still be satisfied, which is a great way to automatically reduce your portion size.)
- Other health benefits include a reduction in diseases of the bowel (including bowel cancer) and reduced cholesterol levels.

Beware Bran As A Source Of Fibre

Two English doctors, Denis Burkitt and Hugh Trowell, alerted the world to the health benefits of high-fibre foods in the 1960s. They had spent many years working in Africa, where they noticed that Africans had a much lower level of diseases such as bowel cancer than Europeans. They linked this to the Africans' very high-fibre diet and made a connection between plenty of fibre and better health. The Africans' source of fibre came from whole grains (not wheat) and fruit. Unfortunately, many people misinterpreted the theory and believed we should add bran to food to increase its fibre content – wheat bran was seen as a convenient source of fibre in the UK because it was readily available and relatively cheap, as it is a by-product of grain milling.

Bran, however, counts as a refined food because it is contained in the grains of cereal plants and then stripped away to be sold on its own. It contains phytates, which have a binding effect on certain vital nutrients such as iron, zinc, calcium and magnesium, making it less easy for the body to absorb them. Eating bran has led to gastrointestinal problems such as bloating and flatulence. It makes much more sense to eat the bran in the form that nature intended by eating the grains in their whole state.

Add Protein To Carbohydrates

Carbohydrates will be broken down into sugar but, as I've already mentioned: the more unrefined the carbohydrate, the slower this happens – with less effect on your blood sugar.

You can change an unrefined carbohydrate into an even slower releasing one by adding protein as you eat it.

So, if you're having porridge, you could add ground nuts and seeds (vegetable protein) and if you are having a jacket potato then you could add tuna (animal protein). You could also sprinkle cinnamon on your porridge, along with the ground nuts and seeds, because cinnamon is helpful in balancing blood sugar, as it improves the transport of glucose into your cells.

Protein slows down the rate at which your stomach empties the food into the next part of the digestive tract and so it slows down the emptying of the carbohydrate too.

If you tend to crave something sweet after a meal, I suggest you add more protein to that meal. When the meal contains a lot of refined starchy carbohydrates, like white rice or white pasta, this will cause your blood sugar to rise quickly. Then, when it drops, you will then crave something sweet. By adding in more protein (say, a piece of fish or nuts and seeds) or substituting a vegetable protein like quinoa for the white rice, you will slow down the rate of digestion and the rise in blood sugar.

Some of your cravings for something sweet after a meal may just be a habit, like always having a biscuit with your cup of tea. Maybe you generally have a dessert after your evening meal or a few squares of chocolate 'to round off the meal' and this has become habitual. So, your body is not actually pushing you to have the sugar because your blood sugar has dropped – but your mind has become used to having something sweet after the meal.

When you feel a craving for something sweet, just take a few moments and give yourself a bit of time to ask how you are really feeling. You may not need that sweet treat after all!

What About A Low Carbohydrate Diet?

As mentioned on page 62, a calorie-restricted diet is not easy for someone to continue long enough to reverse type 2 diabetes, so the better choice seems to be to follow a diet that does not have reduced calories but instead just reduces carbohydrates.

It is now being suggested that lowering carbohydrates should be the first approach to diabetes management.[102] Not only does this way of eating reduce high blood glucose, but it can reduce, or even eliminate, the need for medication and is also easy to follow – especially in the long term.

Research that looked at the benefits of a low carbohydrate diet compared to a calorie-restricted diet over six months for people with type 2 diabetes found that the low carbohydrate diet was effective in lowering HbA1c – but HbA1c didn't decrease in those on the calorie-restricted diet.[103]

And a recent review showed that those who followed a low carbohydrate diet for six months had a remission of diabetes.[104] And what is really interesting is that a low carbohydrate diet that was also high in unsaturated fats (those essential fats on page 118) but low in saturated fats was most beneficial of all. It stabilised blood sugar, reduced the need for diabetes medication and also improved cholesterol (lipid) profiles compared to a high carbohydrate, low fat diet.[105] There was also substantial weight loss, and reduced HbA1c and fasting glucose.

For your diet to count as 'low carbohydrate' your carbohydrate intake needs to be below 130g a day, or less than 26% of 2,000 calories daily.

There have been concerns in the past that a low carbohydrate diet could cause kidney damage, because of the higher volume of protein being processed. And this was thought to be an even bigger concern for someone who already had type 2 diabetes, as this condition often involves some form of kidney damage (caused by high blood sugar levels damaging the blood vessels in the kidneys), without adding to the problem.

But a recent review has shown that patients who had been diagnosed with type 2 diabetes for an average of five years and then followed a low-carb diet over 30 months actually had an improvement in their kidney function.[106] These patients had either normal kidney function or only mild chronic kidney disease, so it is not known yet whether these same improvements in kidney function apply to patients with moderate or severe kidney disease.

It is thought that improving blood sugar levels reduces pressure on the kidneys, so it makes sense to make dietary changes that help improve blood sugar.

I am not suggesting that you follow a low carbohydrate diet in the sense of keeping to 130g per day. I prefer you to aim to eat a lower carbohydrate version of what you would have eaten previously: Reducing or eliminating the amount of refined carbohydrates and including more whole versions, for example swapping white rice for brown rice. And, because you will be adding protein and/or fat to the carbohydrates that you eat, you will automatically be changing the impact that they have on your blood sugar and weight. You are aiming for a way of eating that really becomes a way of life and not a strict low carb diet that you do for a number of months. To help you keep on top of the amount of carbohydrates you are eating, I've included weights for the carbs in the recipes that you can download, see page 179.

Resistant Starch

As the name implies, resistant starch (carbohydrate) means that it resists digestion. It avoids getting digested in the small intestines and ends up fermenting in the large intestines. It is also called fermentable carbohydrate.

Resistant starch is a good thing to include in your diet because these types of carbohydrate are not rapidly converted into glucose (sugar) and so are low on the Glycemic Index. According to the World Health Organisation, resistant starch is the only dietary constituent which shows a convincing protective effect against weight gain.[107]

And, because it is not quickly converted into sugar, it helps to control your blood sugar (glucose) levels[108] and also helps to improve insulin sensitivity.[109]

Foods that contain resistant starch include:

- Legumes like chickpeas, beans and lentils

- Unripe fruit like green bananas

- Wholegrains and seeds (brown rice, barley, wholemeal pasta, oats, wholemeal wheat)

- Cooked, cold food (potatoes, rice, pasta)

There are two forms of starch: amylose and amylopectin. Amylose is the most resistant because it is a tighter molecule and harder for your body to break down. Most starchy carbohydrates will contain a mixture of both amylose and amylopectin.

Legumes have a high content of resistant starch because they have thick cell walls and so make it difficult for the digestive enzymes to break down the starch for digestion.

As we cook foods, this breaks down the cell walls, making the starch more available for digestion so less resistant. But cooking and then cooling the food and eating it cold increases resistant starch content. For example, with potatoes the starch is broken down as the potatoes are cooked but, when left to cool, starch that is formed by the cooling process becomes resistant to digestion.

An easy way to make your bread more GI friendly is to freeze it before you eat it. Whereas the baking process breaks down the starch in wheat and makes it more digestible, when you cool your loaf in the freezer, the starch then becomes resistant. Even if you toast the frozen bread, you will still have a much higher content of resistant starch than if you ate fresh bread.

Starchy Vegetables

Some vegetables have a high amount of carbohydrate and this means that they, too, can raise your blood sugar. Any vegetable with more than five grams (5g) of carbohydrates per 100g of weight is considered to be starchy.

Starchy vegetables which you should limit include:

- Squash
- Sweet potatoes
- Potatoes
- Parsnips
- Sweet corn
- Peas

If you are also having a starchy carbohydrate like rice with your meal try to include non-starchy vegetables. For example:

- Artichoke
- Artichoke hearts
- Asparagus
- Baby corn
- Bamboo shoots
- Bean sprouts
- Beets
- Brussels sprouts
- Broccoli
- Cabbage
- Capsicum (peppers)
- Carrots
- Cauliflower
- Celery

- Coleslaw (no dressing)

- Cucumber

- Courgettes

- Eggplant (aubergines)

- Fennel

- Green beans

- Greens (collard, kale, mustard, turnip)

- Legumes - beans, lentils, chickpeas

- Leeks

- Mushrooms

- Okra

- Onions

- Peppers

- Radishes

- Salad greens (chicory, endive, lettuce, romaine, spinach, radicchio, rocket, watercress)

- Sprouts

- Swiss chard

- Tomato

Fruit

I have mentioned eating whole fruit a few times on previous pages, but it is important to know that it is OK to eat it.

Recent research has shown that people who consume two servings of fruit a day have a 36% lower risk of developing type 2 diabetes over the next five years than those who consume half a serving. (In this study, those who ate more fruit also had better markers of insulin sensitivity, so their bodies produced less insulin to lower their blood sugar levels.) But remember: *fruit juice doesn't count*! You need to eat the whole fruit.[110]

I would be careful with dried fruits like dates because the water has been removed from them and that means the fruit sugar content is much higher than it would be in the fresh fruit. If you are going to eat dried fruit stick to small portions and combine the fruit with a protein such as nuts or seeds.

The best fruits for low GL are cherries, grapefruit, pears, apples, oranges, plums, peaches, grapes and berries, but a handful of nuts or seeds will slow the effect on your bloodstream even more.

Try to minimise the amount of tropical fruits such as bananas, papaya and mangos that you eat. And, if you do want to eat them, try mixing them with low GL fruits in a fruit salad which you can top with yoghurt and/or flaked almonds.

Chapter 13

Our daily bread

"Whether you are having a slice of bread, or a roll, bap, baguette, pitta or bagel – always try to eat a wholegrain version."

Bread is such an iconic food that it's hard to imagine life without it. We 'break bread' with people to show our love and respect for them. We live above or below 'the breadline'. And we 'know which side of our bread is buttered'… Bread is, as another saying goes, 'the staff of life.' It is, for a great many people, a staple food. But it's important to understand the nutritional truth about the type of bread you choose to eat.

• White Bread

White bread is made from wheat that has been stripped of its bran and germ layers, and it may have a longer shelf life because the removal of these parts of the wheat also removes natural oils from the grain. But this means that the fibre is also removed, and one slice of white bread may contain only 0.9g of fibre compared to 2g in a slice of wholemeal bread, and the UK Scientific Advisory Committee on Nutrition say should be aiming for about 30g of fibre a day. (In fact, research has shown that only about 9% of people consume that amount.)[111]

Along with the fibre, vitamins and minerals have also been removed and, in the UK, certain nutrients such as calcium iron, vitamin B2 and vitamin B3 have to be legally added back by the manufacturer. But, as well as the lack of fibre (which is so important for helping to balance your blood sugar), white bread can contain other ingredients (such as sugar, preservatives, flour treatment agents and E numbers) that are not so good for your health. Think about this and read the label on any processed loaf, as you want to improve your diet as much as possible.

• High Fibre White Bread

This is same as the white bread above but here a new source of fibre has been added to the flour. It does seem strange to remove the fibre from the wheat and then add some back in to increase the fibre content, and I don't really consider it a wholefood when parts I want to eat have been removed and replaced with another source of fibre. That said, this loaf will contain more fibre that your usual white bread – and typically 2.6g per slice, which is higher than some wholemeal breads. However, there are also likely to be other, less desirable, ingredients such as sugar, preservatives and E numbers.

• Multigrain Bread

This where I think the terminology becomes confusing because this kind of bread sounds quite 'natural' and wholesome. And yet it is usually made from white flour with added grains, that allow it to be called 'multigrain'. Beware the name, because calling it 'multigrain' does not mean that the grains are in their whole state with a good amount of inherent fibre. It just means that there is a mix of different grains – but these could all be refined. It is clever marketing terminology! A multigrain loaf may also contain seeds, and these could push the fibre content up to about 2g per slice but, again, the bread could contain sugar and flour treatment agents.

• Granary Bread

Again, this one sounds wholesome but it means that the bread contains malted wheat or barley flakes – even though it can be made from white flour. It might be made from wholemeal flour, but you would need to check the label, so don't assume that it is.

• Wholewheat, Wholemeal and Wholegrain Bread

These are basically the same types of bread and include all three parts of the grain; bran, wheatgerm and endosperm.

These breads will naturally contain more fibre and vitamins and minerals than white bread because the grain is whole and has just been milled to make the flour. Again, you will have to check the ingredients as there could be up to 20 or more additives including preservatives, sugar and flour treatment agents.

• Rye Bread

As the name suggests, rye bread is made from rye and it is often heavier than wholewheat bread – but it does make a lovely change. It can be made from the wholegrain so the rye has not been stripped of the fibre and nutrients. Pumpernickel bread is a rye bread traditionally from Germany. It is made from coarsely ground whole rye grains and is often a heavier, denser, flatter type of loaf. I would eat this bread as it is usually quite 'clean', being free of preservatives and flour treatment agents. It contains less gluten than wheat flour and quite a lot of fibre (about 4g per slice), as it is naturally more fibre-rich than wholewheat and contains more nutrients. Studies have shown that rye can help reduce your appetite by helping you to feel full for longer and also slow the release of sugar and insulin into your bloodstream,[112] which of course is so useful for type 2 diabetes. But do still check the ingredient list to see what else has been added to the bread.

• Sourdough

Sourdough has not been made with yeast to make it rise but, instead, a starter culture. This starter is a fermented dough that contains natural yeast and lactic acid bacteria. The starter (sometimes called 'the mother') takes a few days to make and, once it is active, it can be used to keep making sourdough bread (sometimes for years). Any flour can be used to make the bread so it can be made with white flour and will then lack good amounts of fibre, so always read the ingredients on the label. Try to choose a wholemeal sourdough with no additives.

It is thought that sourdough is more easily digested than bread made from yeast due to the sourdough's prebiotic and probiotic qualities from the fermentation and that it causes a lower glycaemic response, making it better for your blood sugar balance.[113]

• Soda Bread

This is a bread from any type of white or wholemeal flour, but sodium bicarbonate is used instead of yeast as the leavening agent. This is a traditional bread in Ireland and also uses buttermilk in the recipe.

• Spelt Bread

Spelt is often called an 'ancient wheat' because it is one of the original strains of wheat. The gluten in spelt is different from the gluten in wheat, in that it is much easier to digest, and a number of people who find wheat a problem can tolerate spelt.

Use Your Loaf...

Bread is a popular, easy and cheap staple of many diets – but if you don't choose your loaf wisely, it can be a wasted opportunity to get the nutrients you need. My recommendation is to eat wholegrain bread where possible so that you get good amounts of fibre, which help to control your blood sugar, along with vitamins and minerals from the whole grains. It doesn't matter whether you are having a slice of bread, or a roll, bap, baguette, pitta or bagel – always try to get a wholegrain version. If you are buying bread for the home, then I would suggest buying organic when you can. It will hopefully contain more naturally-occurring nutrients, because the soil has not been depleted by industrial farming practices. When you eat organically you also avoid pesticide residues which could be detrimental to your general health.

Whether organic or not, always check the ingredients, as you don't want a long list of additives – and you especially don't want sugar.

However, bread isn't for everyone. For those suffering from

Coeliac disease anything containing gluten – a naturally occurring protein in certain grains – is going to be a problem and they will need to eat gluten-free bread which might be made from brown rice, buckwheat, quinoa and/or millet.

Coeliac disease is an autoimmune disease where the gluten in the grain (wheat, barley and rye) triggers the immune system to produce antibodies that, over time, damage the lining of the small intestines. The small villi in the small intestines that absorb nutrients from food end up becoming flattened, and symptoms of Coeliac disease can include diarrhoea, abdominal pain, mouth ulcers, anaemia, skin problems like psoriasis and weight loss.

But it's not only people with Coeliac disease who have a problem with gluten.

Gluten acts like glue. It is stretchy and sticky (think of how a mixture of flour and water is often used as a paste for gluing papier-mâché). The problem is that it has the same effect inside your body, making it hard to digest and that is why some people can experience bloating from eating bread.

Over the years, changes to the way that wheat is bred have intentionally led to an increasingly high gluten content, because this prevents the grain from falling apart as it goes through commercial bakery machines. And we have now come to recognise that you can be sensitive to gluten but not have full-blown Coeliac disease. This has been called '*non-coeliac gluten sensitivity*'. You might have symptoms that are similar to those experienced in Coeliac disease but the antibodies in your blood are negative and gluten is not damaging your small intestines. However, the symptoms of gluten sensitivity can be troubling if you experience them and they include not only gastrointestinal issues like bloating, abdominal discomfort (or pain), diarrhoea and constipation, but also tiredness, lethargy, migraines, headaches and joint pains.

As well as the fact that wheat now contains more gluten than it once did, it has been suggested that these symptoms of gluten sensitivity are a result of bread being made in a much faster way than it was traditionally.

Of course, the more bread that can be made in a shorter space of time, the more commercially viable it is. But the speeding up of this process means there is minimal fermentation – and research has shown that this can cause lower concentrations of good bacteria (bifidobacteria) and more gas than bread made by traditional long fermentation, compared to bread using the Chorleywood breadmaking process.[114]

The Chorleywood breadmaking process shortens the processing time by enabling bread to be produced from the flour, sliced and packaged in roughly three and a half hours. This process also makes a soft fluffy loaf and increases the shelf life. Eighty per cent of bread in the UK is made by this process.

With traditional bread making, the fermentation process alone can take up to three hours and sometimes it is left for 12 hours or more before it is baked. I have had patients who get bloated when eating bread from the supermarkets in the UK – but, when they eat baguettes in France, they feel fine. The same people may also notice that the French baguette is stale the next day – whereas the bread in the UK can last for days.

You could have problems with bread just because you're eating too much of it, too often, in which case see if cutting back helps. But we are all different and have different sensitivities so you could also see how you react to different types of bread. Will sourdough suit you better than a yeasted loaf, for example?

It's also worth remembering to chew really well, because the digestive process starts in your mouth and how the rest of the process goes depends on what happens in your mouth. The digestive enzyme amylase, which is present in your saliva, helps to break down carbohydrates so if these are broken down more efficiently in your mouth, you are going to get less fermentation lower down in your digestive tract and less bloating.

Also, if you want to lose weight, chewing well is really helpful because it takes your brain 20 minutes to register that you are full, so if you take your time and eat slowly you will end up feeling satisfied from eating less. Another useful tip is not to drink with your food. That may mean changing a lifelong habit, but when you drink you dilute those important enzymes in your saliva – so, ideally, don't even drink within 30 minutes either side of a meal.

Chapter 14

Fat matters

"Understand the role that each of the different types of fat plays in your diet."

I've already explained why a low-fat diet can be a bad idea (Chapter 7) – not least because fat is often swapped for sugar in order to add flavour to processed, low fat foods. People have also erroneously come to believe that the healthy antidote to a fatty diet is one that is high in carbohydrates!

However, I am not giving you carte blanche to go off and eat all the fatty foods you like. There are different types of fat – and you need to understand the role that each of these plays in your diet.

Let's start with the one that you must absolutely avoid – and that is a group of fats known as trans fats.

• Trans Fats

Trans fats are the worst fats of all. They have been linked to an increased risk of heart disease and are terrible for your general health. They will cause you to put on more weight around your middle, even if you're sticking to a low-calorie diet[115] – and we know that belly fat is linked to an increased risk of type 2 diabetes. Read your labels and you'll find them (listed as hydrogenated or partially hydrogenated vegetable oil) in many processed foods, such as cakes, biscuits and fast foods – because they're added to prolong these products' shelf life.

They are produced by passing hydrogen through oil at high temperature and under pressure to chemically alter liquid oils to make them into solids. Consuming them is as unnatural to the body as consuming plastic – your body doesn't know what to do with them, so they can cause all sorts of unhealthy processes to occur.

One of these processes is to block the absorption of the essential fatty acids, which your body needs to overcome insulin resistance. So, if you eat trans fats you are hindering any attempts you might be making to improve your insulin sensitivity. To add insult to injury, trans fats harden your insulin receptors (in the same way that they also harden cells and arteries) and this makes you more insulin resistant and encourages your body to produce even higher amounts of insulin. Don't just take my word for it. Studies show that avoiding trans fats can reduce your risk of diabetes by 40%,[116] and research confirms that trans fats can distort cell membranes, and also make their way into your brain cells, altering the ability of your neurons to communicate. Chillingly, scientists have said, 'There is growing evidence for a possible role of trans fats in the development of Alzheimer's disease (type 3 diabetes) and cognitive decline with age.'[117]

Not only do trans fats create more inflammation in your body but, in a horrific double-negative effect, they also block the production of beneficial anti-inflammatory substances. And, although I've shown that fat *per se* is not responsible for high cholesterol levels, trans fats do raise levels of bad cholesterol (LDL), while decreasing levels of good cholesterol (HDL), and therefore increase your risk of heart disease. In fact, if you increase your consumption of trans fats by just two per cent you can increase your risk of heart disease by a massive 30%.[118]

Interestingly, a number of authorities (including those in Denmark, Switzerland, Austria and the city of New York, USA) have banned trans fats – not only in food products but also in restaurants and fast-food outlets. In the UK, officials say a ban would be too difficult to implement, so just be vigilant. Think carefully about whether you really want to eat from a fast food restaurant, and read *all* food labels!

Also, I would suggest you avoid foods labelled 'diabetic' or 'suitable for diabetics'. In fact, since 2016 UK manufacturers have not been allowed to put these words on foods, although they may still be there on food labels in other countries. They were banned in the UK, as the label implied that there were health benefits for people with diabetes to have these foods. Diabetes UK had lobbied for 30 years to have this wording removed from the labels because the foods carrying these words were not any lower in calories and could lead to weight gain, and were usually more expensive.

After trans fats, which I urge you to avoid at all costs, we have saturated and unsaturated fats.

• Saturated Fats

Saturated fats are found in animal products like meat and dairy, and also tropical oils like palm and coconut.

Research has shown that saturated fats can cause insulin resistance and studies looking at red meat consumption in over 140,000 men and women, found that red meat is consistently linked to an increased risk of type 2 diabetes.[119]

However, interesting research on dairy products has shown that yoghurt intake, in particular, is associated with a lower risk of type 2 diabetes.[120] Dairy foods are high in saturated fats but the researchers are thinking that the benefits of the healthy bacteria from fermentation in yoghurt may be a mitigating factor.

People always ask me whether they should use butter or margarine/low-fat spreads. Personally, I choose organic butter as I think it is a more natural product, but I do use it sparingly. Butter is made by churning cream and if you buy an unsalted version there is only one ingredient on the label – butter. A typical margarine could have a list of ingredients including sunflower oil, palm oil, water, salt, emulsifiers, flavour, regulator of acidity, colour, vitamin A, vitamin D. It's also a source of omega 6 fat and I believe most of us have too much of this in our diets (compared to the omega 3 fats we need more of, see Chapter 14).

• Coconut Oil

This deserves a special mention because the nutrition world has changed its view on coconut oil in recent years. Yes, it does contain a high amount of saturated fat (over 90%, which is more than butter), but two thirds of this fat comes in the form of medium chain fatty acids (also known as medium chain triglycerides or MCTs), mainly lauric acid. (Contrast this with dairy products, for example, which only contain about 10 to 12% MCTs.) Lauric acid can easily be converted into energy by the body, instead of being stored as fat. It's also been suggested that coconut oil could help with weight loss because it promotes thermogenesis, the process of increasing metabolism and producing energy.

Coconut oil, like other saturated fats, can be safely used for cooking even at high temperatures. It can't be damaged in the same way as polyunsaturated oils, which, when heated to a high temperature, can create free radicals linked to premature ageing, cancer and heart disease.

• **Unsaturated Fats**

Unsaturated fats include essential fatty acids, which are a vital component of every human cell. Your body needs them to insulate nerve cells, keep your skin and arteries supple, balance hormones and keep you warm.

Essential fatty acids are found in nuts, seeds, beans, oily fish and egg yolks.

Unsaturated fats fall into two main groups: monounsaturated and polyunsaturated.

The mono in monounsaturated fats comes from the fact that, chemically speaking, they only have one double bond. They are known as omega 9 fats and olive oil is high in these fats.

Polyunsaturated fats – as the '*poly*' suggests – can have two or more double bonds and these are *essential* fats because your body cannot produce them. Within this group there is a further split into omega 6 and omega 3 fatty acids, and these oils should have an ideal balance in your body.

Omega 6 oils are found in sunflower, corn, sesame, evening

primrose oil and borage oils. Omega 3s are found in oily fish, flaxseeds (linseeds), soya and walnuts.

• **Omega 3 Essential Fats**

You get omega 3 fatty acids from oily fish, egg yolks, soya, flaxseeds and walnuts and I can't stress enough how important it is to have good levels of them. But there are two issues around omega 3 that you need to understand. The first is that we are not getting enough of it in our diet. The second, and bigger problem, is that we are getting far too much omega 6, and having a higher ratio of omega 6 to 3 creates an inflammatory response in the body.

Omega 6 fats are found in sesame seeds and corn and vegetable oils such as sunflower – and evening primrose oil, which many women have taken for years for PMS. People often take a combined omega 3 and 6 supplement because they have read that we need a good balance of the omega fatty acids. This is true, but you have to take into account what your own levels are in the first place. It is no good adding in more omega 6 if you already have enough, or maybe even too much, in your body.

Signs of a lack of omega 3 fatty acids in your diet include dry skin, lifeless hair, cracked nails, fatigue, depression, dry eyes, lack of motivation, aching joints, difficulty in losing weight, forgetfulness and breast pain. If you have been following the myth that 'fat is fattening', then you could well be deficient in these essential omega 3s, especially if you have followed a low-fat or no fat diet.

We are now getting up to 25 times too much omega 6 from our diet than omega 3.[121] The problem with this imbalance is that having too much omega 6 causes inflammation in your body and it is now thought that inflammation is the underlying cause of all our degenerative diseases including heart disease, cancer, Alzheimer's and type 2 diabetes.

On the other hand, when you eat omega 3 fats, they are converted to substances that have an anti-inflammatory effect in your body. As well as their beneficial anti-inflammatory effects, omega 3 fats can help to balance your blood sugar, by reducing the amount of glucose in your blood, and even switch on anti-diabetic genes.[122] They can also improve levels of a substance called adiponectin which is produced in your fat cells and can regulate glucose. Research is suggesting that this could then reduce the risk of type 2 diabetes and heart disease in people who are obese.[123]

Research in 2021, in a huge analysis of 20 studies from 14 countries including over 65,000 people, showed that those who had good blood levels of EPA (eicosapentaenoic acid) and DHA (docosahexaenoic acid), the two main omega 3s, had a significantly reduced risk of type 2 diabetes.[124] The other form of omega 3, ALA (alpha-linolenic acid), found in flaxseeds, did not show a lower risk.

EPA and DHA are so powerful in helping your cell receptors become sensitive to insulin that one study showed that substituting just seven per cent of dietary fat with omega 3 fatty acids for only four weeks, reversed the need for high levels of insulin to be released in response to a rise in blood sugar.[125]

I would definitely suggest you find out whether you have an imbalance of omega 3 to 6 in your body and how to do this is covered in Chapter 26.

This is important not only in terms of type 2 diabetes and controlling inflammation in obvious places like joints, bowels (e.g. inflammatory bowel disorders) and skin (problems like eczema) but also because research is now pointing out how important these omega 3s are to your brain function and to the prevention of dementia and Alzheimer's.

For your general health, the Harvard School of Public Health has stated that diets deficient in omega 3 cause up to 96,000 preventable deaths a year in the USA.[126] The researchers estimated the number of deaths resulting from 12 preventable causes and omega 3 deficiency ranked as the sixth highest killer of Americans. Conversely, the Framingham Heart Study (one of the longest in the world, following over 240,000 men and 180,000 women over

16 years) found that those with higher levels of omega 3 fat in their blood lived over two years longer than those with lower levels. The researchers found that having low levels of omega 3 was just as strong a predictor of early death as smoking. Also, those people with low omega 3 levels had many different health issues including Alzheimer's and heart disease.[127]

Supplements are a good way to boost your omega 3, but you can also add omega 3 foods, particularly oily fish – sardines, mackerel, salmon, herrings, anchovies and pilchards – into your diet to increase your level. Tuna is also an oily fish but it loses the omega 3 benefit when it is canned, and there are also concerns around eating too much fresh tuna, swordfish and marlin because of the possibility of high mercury levels. It is recommended that there should be maximum intake of four portions of oily fish a week for men and women (past childbearing age). There are no concerns with the supplements, as reputable companies screen the omega 3 content for heavy metals.

Adding oily fish to your diet doesn't have to be expensive or complicated. A recent study found that just adding two cans of sardines in olive oil a week for a year helped to reduce the risk of developing full-blown type 2 diabetes in prediabetic people over the age of 65. They also had increased levels of HDL ('good') cholesterol, reduced insulin resistance and decreased blood pressure.[128] The sardines were added on top of whatever diet the participants were already eating and they were studied against a placebo group too. It was called a sardine-enriched diet but there was no mention of how much oily fish either of the groups might have been eating in the first place.

Excess omega 6 comes from obvious places, such as vegetable oils which are found in a lot of prepared foods. However, a less obvious source of omega 6 fats is from meat and chicken.

You may think you are making a healthier choice by buying corn-fed chicken because it sounds more 'natural'. However, truly free-roaming poultry would feed on a wide variety of foods such as plants, seeds, worms and bugs. Corn-fed chicken only eat corn (which contains high levels of omega 6). As a result, they have lower levels of omega 3 and much higher levels of omega 6 in their meat (and also in their eggs) than chickens allowed to feed in the natural way. A healthy ratio of omega 3 to 6 in eggs would be 1:2 but with corn-fed chickens, eggs can have a ratio of 1:20. There is also the issue of corn-fed chickens being contaminated with pesticides from the corn.

The same issue occurs with grain fed cattle: these, too, give you too much omega 6 and not enough omega 3.[129] In addition, the grain feeding of the cattle causes high level of trans fats. So, eating grain fed beef can increase your risk of heart disease by boosting levels of bad cholesterol (LDL) while decreasing levels of good cholesterol (HDL). ***Remember: If you increase your consumption of trans fats by just two per cent you can increase your risk of heart disease by a massive 30% and these fats can also block the absorption of the essential fats!***[130]

Chapter 15

Choosing an omega 3 supplement

"It is not just the amount of omega 3 contained in your supplement that matters, but the amount of EPA and DHA."

Choosing the right omega 3 supplement can be so complex that I am dedicating a whole chapter to the subject and I hope this will help you navigate your way through the minefield.

The first thing to bear in mind, when you are reading the label of an omega 3 supplement, is that it is not the amount of omega 3 it contains that matters, but the amount of EPA (eicosapentaenoic acid) and DHA (docosahexaenoic acid). Unless you are vegetarian or vegan, take an omega 3 fish oil supplement containing 770mg EPA and 510mg DHA (the one I use in my clinic is NHP's Omega 3 Support www.naturalhealthpractice.com).

If you are vegan or vegetarian, look for vegan EPA and DHA from algae. Other plant sources of omega 3, such as walnuts, chia and flaxseeds, provide ALA (alpha-linolenic acid) which your body has to convert into EPA and DHA – but this is not a very satisfactory process, and it is thought that there may only be a five to 10% conversion from ALA to EPA and DHA. That's a problem, because EPA and DHA significantly reduce your risk of type 2 diabetes – but the ALA found in flaxseeds, etc. does not.[131]

I don't use any cod liver oil supplements in my clinics, because the oil extracted from the liver of the fish (rather than the body) can contain high quantities of heavy metals or toxins. In 2006, in the UK two companies had to remove their cod liver oil capsules from the shelves because they contained toxic dioxins (a carcinogen) at a level above the legal limit.

When you're choosing an omega 3 supplement, therefore, check that the oils come from the body of the fish and try and make sure that the supplement you choose comes from wild rather than farmed fish and small fish, such as anchovies and sardines. Large fish, such as tuna, can contain high levels of mercury.

As well as the amount of EPA and DHA, check the form of the omega 3 oil as there are three main forms with important differences.

- Phospholipids

- Ethyl esters

- Triglycerides

Below, I look at omega 3 supplements taken from krill, which comes in the phospholipid form. I don't advise taking this kind of omega 3 supplement; read on to see why. Ethyl ester forms of omega 3 fish oil are synthetic and based in alcohol. They are the cheapest form of fish oil to produce, but they are also the least bioavailable. As your body usually ingests fats in the triglyceride form, an oil in the ethyl ester form has to be converted back into a triglyceride.

Research has shown that the triglyceride fish oils are better absorbed than the ethyl ester forms. Ethyl esters are also less stable than triglyceride fish oils and so can oxidise, creating free radicals in your body.

This means, then, that the triglyceride is the most natural form – it is the form in which you would absorb omega 3 oils from eating the fish. In fact, more than 98% of all fats are triglycerides.

I must mention krill oil because there has been such media hype about it. As I've said, when you eat fish, you absorb the omega 3 fat in the triglyceride form. Those who advocate krill oil supplementation claim that it is superior to fish oil because it comes in the phospholipid form, which manufacturers say the body finds easier to absorb.

A study in 2013 suggested that krill oil could be more effective than fish oil at improving omega 3 levels and reducing the omega 6 to omega 3 ratio.[132] Then, in 2014, researchers said that the study was flawed, because the scientists did not use a typical fish oil (which is high in omega 3), but an oil high in omega 6 fatty acids, skewing the results.

Other scientists made this comment: 'Due to the fatty acid profile being non-representative of typically commercially marketed fish oil, the conclusions presented by Ramprasath et al are not justified and [are] misleading. Considerable care is needed in ensuring that such comparative trials do not use inappropriate ingredients.'[133]

The EPA and DHA in krill oil supplements is very low. For about 2,000mg krill you get around 240mg EPA and 110mg DHA. The same amount of fish oil supplement gives about 770mg EPA and 510mg DHA. Still further controversy arrived in 2014 when research re-examined the studies which have looked at the bioavailability of krill oil – that is how easily krill oil is absorbed into your body. They point out that it has proven difficult to compare the bioavailability of krill oil versus fish oil, because of the lower concentrations of both EPA and DHA in krill oil compared to fish oil. They also point to other factors that have made it difficult to compare the two and conclude 'that there is at present no evidence for greater bioavailability of krill oil versus fish oil'.[134]

It wasn't until the scientists designed a study comparing krill to fish oil using the same amount of EPA and DHA that we could see that, as long as you compared like with like, then you got similar rises in blood levels of EPA and DHA.[135] But you would need to take at least three times as much of the krill oil to match the levels of EPA and DHA in fish oil.

One well known supplement company who sells krill oil has now 'fortified' (their words) their krill oil supplement with fish oil on their 'nutritionists' advice'. To me, it just makes more sense to take fish oil in the first place.

Finally, my last concern about krill oil is an ecological one. Krill is not a fish, but a crustacean and it is the bottom of the food chain for many animals, including whales, fish, seals and seabirds. It seems that the whole Antarctic ecosystem revolves around it. Some health food stores have taken krill oil off the shelves because of the decline in certain sea animals, whales, penguins and seals where the krill is harvested.

The Bottom Line

Look for an omega 3 supplement that provides daily amounts of around 770mg EPA and 510mg DHA, whether from a fish source or a vegan algae omega 3 supplement.

Chapter 16

You are what you drink

"Still or sparkling water is your healthiest option."

We've covered soft drinks and know that both sugared and artificially sweetened drinks risk raising your blood sugar level and also causing you to gain weight. But what about other drinks? Could they also increase your risk of type 2 diabetes?

• Caffeine

Could coffee be helpful for diabetes? As always, there can be conflicting studies – with some research showing that coffee could accelerate the development of type 2 diabetes by reducing insulin sensitivity and raising fasting insulin levels,[136] while other research has suggested that three cups of tea or coffee a day could actually reduce your risk by 40%.[137]

When research comes up with such contradictory results, it's hard to know what to do, and who to believe. Dig a little deeper, though, and the participants in the first study had actually increased their coffee consumption very quickly over four weeks. That could have led to the detrimental effect on insulin sensitivity. Another possibility was that the participants' increased stress levels may have been responsible. I think this last point is really important. Caffeine consumption might be helpful for type 2 diabetes treatment and prevention, but I would be very wary of consuming high amounts if you are stressed. Caffeine is a stimulant that can make you feel more stressed – and we know that being stressed causes your blood to hang on to glucose, meaning that you become less sensitive to insulin.

As ever, moderation is key – but your individual circumstances will also determine whether or not coffee is right for you, if you're concerned about type 2 diabetes or have already been diagnosed with it.

In other research, looking at whether coffee could be helpful for non-alcoholic fatty liver disease, coffee drinkers were found to be 39% less likely to develop cirrhosis.[138] Chemicals in coffee are converted into paraxanthine, a compound that slows the growth of scar tissue, and two other chemicals in coffee – kahweol and cafestol – may also prevent liver cancer.

• Alcohol

It's important to think about different types of alcohol and whether they have a higher or lower sugar content, because they will have an effect on your blood sugar. Red wine is thought to be one of the healthiest alcoholic drinks because of its high content of antioxidants, but you could also have white wine and make it into a spritzer by adding mineral water, so you end up drinking less alcohol. Also, the drier the wine, the less sugar, so a dry white is a better option than a sweeter one. Fortified wines, such as sherry and port, are high in sugar.

Spirits are considered 'better' because they do not contain sugar – but do think about the sugar content of your choice of mixer drink, and avoid the soft drinks I've already discussed in earlier chapters. Still or sparkling water is your healthiest option.

Beer contains a lot of carbohydrate, which can cause weight gain – hence the term 'beer belly'.

And, needless to say, liqueur spirits such as Cointreau, Cherry Brandy and Drambuie contain a lot of sugar.

• Fruit Juice

It might surprise you to learn that fruit juice is classed as a refined carbohydrate because the juicing process removes most of the fibre, which remains in the wasted pulp. This means that the natural sugars in the fruit flow into the juice without any moderating fibre. When you drink juice, the sugars hit your blood stream quickly, forcing your pancreas to pump out a lot of insulin.

With this in mind, it's important to limit fruit juices when you are working on preventing or treating type 2 diabetes. Whole fruit, with all its fibre intact, is a much better option. In fact, one large long-term study found that increasing fruit and vegetable consumption **reduced** the risk of diabetes but increasing fruit juice consumption by just one serving a day gave an 18% **increased** risk of diabetes.[139]

It would be better to eliminate fruit juice completely but, if you are going to drink it, dilute it half and half with water so that it is not so concentrated – and don't drink juice on an empty stomach as it is going to hit your bloodstream very quickly. Remember that, as I've already said elsewhere, a single glass of orange juice can contain the juice of up to eight oranges and you would never eat that amount of whole oranges in one go, and that is a lot of fruit sugar. A smoothie is slightly better than a juice as it is just the food blended up without the loss of fibre – but it will still be absorbed faster than if you had sat down and chewed all those fruits and vegetables as whole foods because the smoothie is a liquid.

Finally, avoid anything called 'fruit juice drink', which is likely to contain refined sugar or artificial sweeteners.

• Water

Whatever else you are drinking, and however you are trying to keep it safe, do remember to make sure you are drinking enough water – because just allowing yourself to become dehydrated is enough to trigger high blood sugar!

It makes sense that, if you don't have good fluid intake, the sugar in your circulation can become more concentrated. But this also causes you to urinate more, and the more you urinate, the more dehydrated you will be... So, you can quickly become caught in a vicious cycle.

Many people deliberately limit the amount of water that they drink – for fear that they will want to urinate when they know it's going to be inconvenient. But, in fact, they are risking the chain reaction of dehydration and high blood sugar which will, ironically, make them want to pee more.

Dehydration causes the release of a hormone called vasopressin, which is an anti-diuretic hormone to stop you losing water. It controls the amount of urine your kidneys produce. When you are dehydrated, your pituitary gland releases vasopressin and, in response, your kidneys will stop the production of urine.

Because vasopressin is regulating fluid control it also has an impact on raising blood pressure. Diuretics, also known as 'water pills', are often used to help control high blood pressure by aiming to help your kidneys produce more urine.

As well as controlling dehydration, vasopressin has been shown to play a role in blood sugar balance and high levels of the hormone are linked to diabetes.[140] It's a vicious cycle with drinking too little water increasing your risk of diabetes, and diabetes increasing your risk of dehydration, as high blood glucose causes you to be more dehydrated!

If your blood sugar stays high for too long a period of time, your kidneys will aim to remove the excess glucose from the blood and pass this out through the urine. Because your kidneys are filtering the blood to remove the extra glucose, they are also removing water. So, if you notice you are passing urine more often but also feeling thirsty, this could be a sign that your blood sugar level is too high and causing you to become dehydrated.

As well as having a dry mouth, your urine would be a dark yellow colour when you are dehydrated. Your urine is often darker in the morning when you have first got up, as it has become concentrated overnight, but it shouldn't stay that way during the day.

The recommendation is to drink at least one and a half litres (six to eight glasses) of water a day. It has been suggested that this could be calculated according to your size. Taking your weight in pounds and halving that figure should tell you how much water in ounces you should drink in a day. But you may need to increase your water intake beyond this amount if you drink tea, coffee, caffeinated fizzy drinks and alcohol – all of which will dehydrate your body. You also need to drink more if you are exercising a lot, travelling by plane, eating a lot of salty foods, or you're in a hot environment. Conversely, if you're eating a lot of fruit and vegetables, you will not need so much extra water as these can contain up to 90% water.

If you're not a fan of plain water, remember that herbal teas count towards your daily intake as they are caffeine-free, so won't dehydrate you. You could also add a slice of lemon or some fresh mint leaves to hot or cold water to make it more palatable, and frozen berries also make a refreshing drink in cold water.

Water, Water, Everywhere

- Your body is two-thirds water, and this is what provides the means for nutrients to travel to organs and for toxins to be removed.

- It also helps your body metabolise stored fat, so it is crucial for weight management.

- Water is lost through urination, respiration and sweating, and symptoms of mild dehydration include joint pain, irritability, headache, tension, swollen ankles and a bloated stomach.

- A strong odour to your urine, along with a yellow or amber colour can also be an indicator of dehydration – and will often occur before your body registers that it needs water and you start to feel thirsty.

- Sometimes you might think you're feeling hungry when really what you're experiencing is thirst. Drinking a glass of water and waiting 20 minutes will tell you if you really do need to eat something and will help you avoid unnecessary snacking.

Chapter 17

Know your nutrients

"Investing in the best quality supplements you can afford will help you turn your health around as quickly as possible."

You might think that you can get all the nutrition you need from a 'well-balanced diet'. Indeed, many doctors reinforce this message. But what does a 'well-balanced diet' really mean? There is no agreed definition – and when you are trying to correct or prevent a health problem, certain nutrients are going to be especially beneficial, so you really need to know that your diet is giving you what you need.

The problem is that over-farming and the use of pesticides mean much of the soil our food is grown in has become depleted in vital nutrients. Many supermarket fruit and vegetables have travelled hundreds of miles over many days to get to the shelves, with meagre nutrients becoming ever more depleted as the gap between being picked and being sold widens.

Today's fruit and vegetables typically contain about 20% fewer minerals than they did in the 1930s. Magnesium is down by 24%, calcium by 46%, iron by 27%, and zinc by 59%. Iron levels in modern meat are down by 47%, in milk by over 60%, and calcium levels in cheese are down by 15% (and Parmesan cheese by 70%).[141]

All this means that many people are now quite deficient in certain vitamins and minerals as well as omega 3 essential fatty acids. This is especially likely to be true among people who have dieted in the past. It is possible, and increasingly common, to be overfed yet undernourished – and this is what happens when you eat more than you need – and enough to cause you to put on weight – but if the bulk of your diet is highly processed and refined.

Fascinating research from 2020 looked at the food diaries of people who were overweight or obese and found that, although they appeared to be getting enough nutrients from their food, when their blood was tested most of the participants were severely deficient in vitamins A and D, calcium, potassium, magnesium and zinc.[142] This suggests that eating too much can be a sign that your body lacks nutrients, and it is trying to compensate by getting you to eat more.

My recommendation would be to make all the dietary recommendation in Chapter 7 and then follow a specific programme of supplements for at least six months.

In my clinics I test patients to assess specific nutrient deficiencies (see Chapter 26) but, even without being tested, you can start to make a difference to your health with specific nutrients and herbs that we know are key to helping manage or prevent type 2 diabetes. Do remember, though, that supplements can never be a substitute for the dietary recommendations. The clue is in the name: supplements are 'supplementary' to your food and no excuse to move away from a healthy way of eating. However, they will certainly help with type 2 diabetes and also improve your general health.

Supplements

I always recommend my patients buy the best quality supplements they can afford, because these are likely to contain higher doses of nutrients than cheap supplements, and in forms that are more easily absorbed by the body. It really is worth making that investment if you want to turn your health around as quickly as possible.

When you're trying to choose between the many options available, capsules are always better than tablets because your body doesn't have to work so hard to get at the nutrients (it merely has to melt the capsule, rather than try to break down a compressed tablet which contains binders to hold the nutrients together). It's also a good idea to avoid chewable or fizzy tablets as these are usually packed with unwanted ingredients such as colourings, sugar, or artificial sweeteners, which may even add to your problems.

You only want the active ingredients, like the vitamins and minerals that you want the supplement for. But even capsules can have added ingredients that you may not have previously come across. These are called *excipients* and are non-active ingredients with no nutritional value to you but they are added to the supplement for the manufacturer's benefit, not yours. They are lubricants, anti-caking agents, disintegrants, fillers or bulking agents which make the supplements faster and easier to manufacture – and, therefore, cheaper and more profitable for the companies to make. Excipients can include magnesium stearate, titanium dioxide, talc, calcium hydrogen phosphate dehydrate, stearic acid.

Without lubricants and anti-caking agents, the manufacturing process has to be slowed down to allow the nutrients to flow into the capsules. When the machinery is slowed down, less heat is generated and this is beneficial when dealing with natural ingredients like herbs and enzymes. But doing this actually presents a huge challenge for a lot of manufacturers so most supplement companies on the market will just have these non-active, non-nutrients added into the capsules.

But think about it: when these excipients are added to the supplements, there is less space for the active nutrients because the lubricants and anti-caking agents are taking up that space – and, as there's no requirement to list the amount of excipients in the supplement, you have no way of knowing what proportion of your capsule, tablet or pill is the inactive ingredients compared to the active nutrients that you really want.

Your Type 2 Diabetes Supplement Programme

An analysis of 108 clinical trials using supplements on over 4,000 patients with diabetes or poor glucose control showed an improvement in the control of blood sugar in more than 75% of cases[143] – so supplements definitely have a role to play as you go forward.

See below for my recommended supplement programme, along with detailed information about each supplement and required dosages. I will cover each nutrient separately to show its benefits and the research that supports these, but I would always suggest that you take combinations of nutrients. Over the last 30 years or more that I have been in clinical practice, I have found that combinations – whether nutrients or herbs – are more powerful and effective than single nutrients on their own.

When you eat, you are consuming a number of different nutrients together and many of them will work synergistically, helping each other to become more effective. Nutrients in supplement form work in the same way – used in the right combinations, they are more beneficial than when they are taken individually. For example, research has shown that magnesium is more effective for people with severe stress[144] when it's taken with vitamin B6 than when it's taken on its own.

For type 2 diabetes, I recommend taking a good combination supplement containing chromium, all the B vitamins, zinc, manganese, magnesium, Q10, alpha lipoic acid, biotin, inositol, carnitine, folic acid (as folate), vitamin D3, N acetyl cysteine and cinnamon (see Chapter 19) (NHP's Blood Sugar (Glucose) Support which contains all these nutrients is available at www.naturalhealthpractice.com), together with additional vitamin C and probiotic and omega 3 fish oil supplements (which are discussed in Chapters 18 and 15).

• Chromium

The most widely studied nutrient in blood sugar control,[145] and the most important nutrient for type 2 diabetes, chromium helps to balance your blood sugar, improves insulin resistance, reduces food cravings and also aids weight loss. By improving the action of insulin, it enables glucose to move out of the blood so that it can be used by cells for energy. But, without chromium, insulin is less effective at controlling blood sugar levels and glucose levels rise.

The bad news is that too few people have enough chromium in

their diet. The mineral should be naturally present in grains such as oats, rice, wheat, corn and rye. However, as soon as these grains are refined (turned into white bread, pastries, biscuits and even pasta) the chromium is stripped out. It's a vicious circle: chromium is vital to keep blood sugar in balance but is not present in refined food – and refined food is part of the cause of the blood sugar imbalance.

Chromium is also the most widely researched mineral for the treatment of obesity – partly because it helps to control cravings and reduces hunger. In one eight-week trial, healthy overweight women who took chromium supplements ate less, felt less hungry, craved less and lost more weight than those taking a placebo.[146]

If you are already insulin resistant, chromium can help by making your body's cells more sensitive to insulin – and research has shown that the lower someone's levels of chromium, the more likely they are to have problems with glucose and insulin regulation. People with type 2 diabetes have been found to have low levels of chromium[147] but taking chromium (combined with biotin, see below) will improve your blood sugar control.

As an added bonus, chromium has also been found to help break down fat and cholesterol in the blood – and a deficiency has not only been linked to high blood glucose but also to high cholesterol and the development of plaque in the arteries.[148]

Take: 200mcg chromium per day

• Zinc

After chromium, I always recommend zinc to help control sugar cravings and blood sugar swings. It's another nutrient that helps insulin to work more effectively, and it can also optimise your sense of taste and smell,[149] which helps with appetite control. If you are not experiencing the full taste of your food, it is harder to appreciate the more subtle sweetness in foods – and that can lead you to crave and eat refined sugars to get a stronger taste.

Another way that zinc manages appetite is by increasing levels of leptin, the hormone that tells you when you feel satisfied and have had enough to eat. This is particularly important if you feel you always want something sweet after a meal.[150]

As well as helping with blood sugar control, zinc has a widespread beneficial effect on your general health. It's well known for improving immune function, but it is also needed to produce stress hormones, insulin and sex hormones, and is crucial for maintaining healthy liver and immune function. In fact, it's needed for about 200 different enzyme processes in your body, and for healthy cell division.

If you are deficient in zinc, insulin cannot do its job properly and glucose cannot enter the cells. Because insulin levels then remain high in the blood, more insulin will be produced, leading to insulin resistance over time.

Zinc, together with selenium, has been found to be lower in women with gestational diabetes, so these are important minerals during pregnancy.[151]

Take: 10mg zinc per day

• Biotin

Biotin is part of the B vitamin family and, when combined with chromium, it helps balance blood sugar and aids the metabolism of carbohydrates. Biotin is also involved in the production of glucose and the effective use of it.

Working synergistically with insulin, it is involved in many enzyme reactions in the body, some which are also related to blood sugar level. Research on animals has shown that using chromium and biotin together could potentially be more beneficial for the treatment of insulin resistance and the prevention of diabetes than using either nutrient separately.[152]

Take: 35mcg biotin per day

• Alpha Lipoic Acid

Alpha lipoic acid helps insulin to move glucose into your cells and, therefore, plays an important role in both the prevention and treatment of diabetes.[153] Research has shown that, as well as preventing insulin resistance, it can prevent high blood pressure.[154] It also helps to support healthy liver function and, because it is such a powerful antioxidant, it can slow down the ageing process.

If you have neuropathy, it's worth knowing that alpha lipoic acid works quicker and is better tolerated than licensed painkillers for treating symptoms of this serious complication of diabetes, such as numbness, muscle strength, paraesthesia (pins and needles) and pain.[155]

Take: 100mg alpha lipoic acid per day

• Carnitine

The amino acid carnitine's role is to break down fat to release energy. It's been shown to lower triglycerides (blood fats), increase HDL ('good') cholesterol and reduce LDL ('bad') cholesterol. Studies have found that it may improve insulin sensitivity in patients with type 2 diabetes[156] and also that low levels are connected to a number of diabetic complications.[157]

Take: 200mg carnitine per day

• Co-enzyme Q10

This essential vitamin-like substance is contained in nearly every cell in your body.

One of its roles is to break down carbohydrates and turn them into energy so they are not stored as fat – but it also helps your body to burn fat for energy. A deficiency in co-enzyme Q10, which becomes more likely as you get older, actually makes you age faster, accelerating DNA damage, and also depleting your energy levels – the reason that supplements are often recommended to treat fatigue.

Co-enzyme Q10 helps to lower glucose and insulin, so it has a role to play in controlling blood sugar levels, reversing insulin resistance, and helping with glycaemic control in people with type 2 diabetes. And it also helps to improve blood pressure[158] (one of your other risk factors, alongside type 2 diabetes, for metabolic syndrome, see page 18). When, in a randomised double-blind trial, co-enzyme Q10 was given to patients with high blood pressure who were already taking blood pressure medication, the patients achieved lower levels of both glucose and insulin as well as lower blood pressure and lower levels of triglycerides (blood fats).[159] Their HDL ('good' cholesterol) increased as did their levels of antioxidants, vitamins A, C, E and beta carotene.

Co-enzyme Q10 is a particularly important nutrient to take if you are on statins, as these not only reduce your liver's production of cholesterol but also reduce the production of co-enzyme Q10. In fact, just two weeks on a statin can cause a significant decrease in co-enzyme Q10 levels.[160] But, by supplementing this nutrient, it is also possible to offset some of the muscle-related side effects connected with statins.[161]

Do talk to your doctor if you are on statins and are also worried about your blood sugar because, unfortunately, statins can increase your risk of developing type 2 diabetes by almost 50%.[162] They decrease insulin sensitivity by 24% and also reduce the pancreas's ability to secrete insulin by 12%.

Take: 25mg co-enzyme Q10 per day

• Inositol

Inositol is a B vitamin and is found naturally in a number of foods including beans, grains, nuts and fruit. Your body can also produce it from the carbohydrates you eat.

It can be helpful in regulating blood sugar, improving fasting blood glucose and also lowering HbA1c.[163] And there is research to show that it can also be effective in the prevention and treatment of both type 2 diabetes and gestational diabetes.[164]

Take: 50mg inositol per day

• Manganese

Manganese helps to maintain a healthy blood sugar balance by stimulating glycogen storage in your liver. It also has a role to play in metabolism and healthy thyroid function, and in helping your body to properly utilise vitamin C and the B vitamins.

A large study of over 84,000 postmenopausal women without a history of diabetes found that those who had higher intakes of manganese had a lower risk of type 2 diabetes.[165]

Interestingly, if guinea pigs (which, like us humans, do not manufacture their own vitamin C) become manganese deficient they develop diabetes.

Take: 5mg manganese per day

• Magnesium

Known as 'nature's tranquilliser', because it calms your adrenal glands, magnesium also helps to balance blood sugar by contributing to the production and action of insulin – and there is a strong link between being deficient in magnesium and insulin resistance.[166]

But the higher your magnesium levels the greater your sensitivity to insulin (which is a good thing). One older study of 12,000 people over the course of six years showed that people with the lowest intake of magnesium had a 94% chance of developing type 2 diabetes[167] while newer research on 17,000 people, over 28 years, showed that those with the highest magnesium intake had a 15% lower risk of type 2 diabetes than those with the lowest intake.[168]

The evidence is suggesting that supplementing with magnesium can delay the progress to type 2 diabetes if you have been diagnosed with prediabetes.[169] This is so important if you have been diagnosed with prediabetes and you are working on reversing it.

Take: 40mg magnesium per day

• B Vitamins

The B vitamins are known as the 'anti-stress' vitamins, and they are all needed for food to be turned into energy rather than body fat.

Vitamin B3 helps to release energy from carbohydrates and works with chromium to balance blood sugar.

Vitamin B6 is needed for energy production and the metabolism of essential fatty acids.

Folic acid is another important B vitamin and, along with vitamins B6 and B12, it helps to control a substance called homocysteine. This is a toxic by-product from the breakdown of methionine (one of the essential amino acids) and it should, under normal circumstances, be detoxified (broken down and excreted) by the body.

High levels of homocysteine have been linked to heart disease, Alzheimer's and osteoporosis, and research has also looked at whether there is a link between high homocysteine levels and high levels of insulin. In one study, people with metabolic syndrome (see page 18) were given both folic acid and B12. This combination not only reduced homocysteine levels, as one would expect, but it also had a positive effect on insulin resistance. It seems that the lower the level of homocysteine, the lower the level of insulin.[170] But make sure you take folic acid in the active form of methylfolate. This is closest to the form you'd get naturally from food – and nowadays you can get supplements where the folic acid is in the methylfolate form and not the synthetic folic acid form.

Everybody knows that folic acid is important for a healthy pregnancy and newborn – because it helps prevent neural tube defects, such as spina bifida, in the baby. And, as we have seen, it is important, together with vitamins B6 and vitamin B12, to lower circulating levels of homocysteine.

When you take folic acid in supplement form, your body converts it to l-methylfolate. However, some people have a genetic variation that makes it difficult for them to make the conversion. So, it is better to have folic acid in the active methylfolate form to make sure your body can use it effectively.

Take: 10-25mg of most of the B vitamins per day

• Vitamin D

Vitamin D is your 'sunshine vitamin' and it has been known for many years that it is important for bone health and the prevention of osteoporosis, because you need good levels of this vitamin in order to absorb calcium, and to make sure that calcium ends up in your bones and is not deposited somewhere else in your body, such as in your joints (calcification).

But research into the benefits of vitamin D has exploded over the past 20 years and we now know that it plays a major role in breast and bowel cancer prevention as well as immune function, autoimmune diseases, heart disease, joint pains and arthritis, dementia, fertility, autism and allergies. And of course, type 2 diabetes.

Natural food sources of vitamin D are few – mainly oily fish and eggs. One hundred grams of grilled salmon contains 284iu of vitamin D and 100g of tinned pilchards contains 560iu of vitamin D, the yolk of one egg contains about 20iu of vitamin D.

There is some concern that most people today are not getting much vitamin D from their diet, especially those who are eating junk food and not eating any, or very little, oily fish or eggs, and scientists are noting a rise in the bone disease rickets in children who are not eating enough vitamin D rich foods and are spending too little time outdoors.

You manufacture vitamin D through your skin during exposure to sunlight, so you're most at risk of a deficiency if you don't go out much in the daytime, or don't expose your skin to the sunlight, for example if your make-up or cosmetics contain sun protection factors (SPFs). It is estimated that we need about 30 minutes exposure to the sun daily to produce enough vitamin D.

Vitamin D is now recognised as being very important for controlling blood sugar and improving insulin sensitivity,[171] and research is now suggesting that having good levels of vitamin D can help to prevent type 2 diabetes[172] with those with the highest vitamin D status (greater than 62.5nmol/l (25ng/ml)) having a 43% lower risk of developing type 2 diabetes compared to those with the lowest level (less than 35nmol/l (14ng/ml)).[173]

Since I've already mentioned the effect that statins for cholesterol can have on insulin, it's also important to know that your body uses cholesterol to make vitamin D, and – if your vitamin D level is low – your body can end up producing more cholesterol in order to manufacture more vitamin D. By correcting a vitamin D deficiency, your cholesterol level could go down, reducing your need for statins.

Also, if you are overweight, with a higher percentage of body fat, this can 'steal' vitamin D from your blood – and a vitamin D deficiency is much more common in overweight people.

But, as always with Nature, there is a need for balance. You don't want to be deficient in vitamin D but nor do you want to overload your body with it. Lately it has become fashionable to take mega doses of vitamin D. It is a fat-soluble nutrient so you can store it in your body, unlike vitamin C which is water-soluble. And, because it can be stored, it can become toxic if levels become too high.

Having a level of vitamin D below 10nmol/l (4ng/ml) increases your risk of dying from any cause (known as 'all-cause mortality'). But a level above 140nmol/ (56ng/ml) also increases your risk of dying from any cause.[174]

My recommendation is to do a simple home finger prick test for vitamin D (Chapter 26) so you know whether or not you are deficient. If your levels are low, I recommend adding in a separate vitamin D supplement for three months (on top of your multivitamin and mineral) and then re-testing to make sure that the level is back to normal (for information on organising the vitamin D test see Resources page 240). And make sure that you are taking vitamin D3 and not D2. D3 is 87% more effective at raising and maintaining vitamin D levels than D2.[175]

Take: 800iu of vitamin D per day

• N-Acetyl Cysteine

N-acetyl cysteine (NAC) is a form of the amino acid cysteine and is another powerful antioxidant. Adding this to your diet as a supplement will help reduce insulin levels and make your body more sensitive to insulin, research shows.[176] And research on animals has shown that NAC could help to prevent the development of prediabetes and inflamed liver problems.[177]

NAC has been shown to be helpful in protecting you against diabetes-related heart complications if you have already been diagnosed with type 2 diabetes.[178] Up until recently, heart failure was the leading cause of death in people with diabetes (that has now been overtaken by cancer) and there was no treatment to protect you against the risk of developing cardiovascular complications. But, because of its antioxidant benefits, NAC can help by preventing cardiac damage and the risk of heart attack (myocardial infarction). It can also help to remove heavy toxic metals like mercury, lead and cadmium from the body by binding to them and pulling them out.

Take: 500mg N-acetyl cysteine per day

• Vitamin C

Everyone tends to associate vitamin C with immune system function and also its antioxidant benefits. But it is an unusual nutrient in that most animals can make vitamin C from glucose, but we humans can't. We have to get enough vitamin C from our diet or from supplements.

Vitamin C and glucose are very similar in their molecular structure and use the same transport systems in your body so they can end up competing with each other. If you have high levels of glucose (sugar) in your blood you can end up with low levels of vitamin C, as the vitamin C will not be able to get into your cells – and both glucose and vitamin C need insulin to get into your cells via insulin receptors.

Glucose always takes priority, as it has a stronger affinity for these insulin receptors than vitamin C, and this means that the higher your blood glucose (sugar), the less vitamin C will make it into your cells.

The good news is that research has shown that giving a total of 1,000mg of vitamin C a day to people with type 2 diabetes reduces both fasting blood sugar levels and HbA1c. The vitamin C also reduces LDL ('bad' cholesterol). It is interesting that 500mg of vitamin C a day was not enough to reduce fasting blood sugar, HbA1c or LDL.[179]

Vitamin C can also be helpful for Alzheimer's (which is now being thought of as type 3 diabetes), with research on mice showing that vitamin C supplementation can reduce the beta-amyloid plaque build-up[180] that causes this disease. There is also research suggesting that the breaking down of the blood–brain barrier is a factor in the progression of Alzheimer's disease, and we know that vitamin C helps to maintain the integrity of the barrier between your blood and brain.

Vitamin C can also be helpful if you're trying to lose weight to help prevent or reverse type 2 diabetes or prediabetes; and that is because having good levels of vitamin C enables you to burn 30% more fat when you're doing moderate exercise than you would if you had low levels of the vitamin.[181] It is thought that when vitamin C levels are low, the body slows down fat burning as a safety measure.

I would suggest that you take 1,000mg of vitamin C, split into two lots of 500mg. The split is important as vitamin C is a water-soluble nutrient, so you lose it through your urine during the day. Make sure you are taking the alkaline form of vitamin C (as magnesium ascorbate) rather than the acidic form (ascorbic acid). The alkaline form is much gentler on your digestive system and it will be clear on the label as to what form the vitamin C is.

NHP's Vitamin C Support is my recommendation (www.naturalhealthpractice.com).

Take: 500mg vitamin C twice per day

More About The Benefits Of Vitamin D...

- It is an immune modulator, meaning it balances your immune function, helping to boost your immunity if it's running low, but also helping to dampen it down if it becomes overactive, as happens with autoimmune conditions (such as rheumatoid arthritis and lupus).

- It promotes apoptosis, the body's way of eliminating unhealthy cells which could otherwise continue to survive.

- It can help fight cancer. Studies show it can stop the multiplication of malignant breast cells,[182] halve the risk of developing cancer,[183] and reduce cancer mortality by 13%.[184]

  - It controls inflammation by increasing levels of substances which are anti-inflammatory at the same time as reducing those that cause inflammation. If you are having severe joint and even muscle pains (which can be a sign of inflammation), I would suggest that you have a blood test for vitamin D (see page 229) and supplement with extra if needed. Research has shown that once you correct the deficiency the pain goes away.[185]

The Bottom Line

My recommendation, then, is to take a good supplement programme. I have formulated a supplement for NHP called Blood Sugar (Glucose) Support which contains all the nutrients mentioned above including cinnamon (see Chapter 19) and take additional supplements of vitamin C, omega 3 and a probiotic (which are discussed in Chapters 15 and 18).

PART 3

BOOST YOUR HEALTH

Chapter 18

Meet your gut microbiome

"Our probiotic health actually affects nearly every aspect of our wellbeing."

Over the last few years, research into our gut microbiome has exploded. We now know far more than we did only a few years ago about the importance of the vast forest of healthy bacteria (probiotics) contained in our gut, and how they benefit our health. And, our greater understanding has shown us that these benefits go way beyond the gut and that our probiotic health actually affects nearly every aspect of our wellbeing.

Scientists talk about the brain–gut axis; and they even call the gut the 'second brain', because it is filled with the same neurotransmitters as your brain. Therefore, what is good for your gut is also good for your brain, and your probiotic health has direct effects on your memory, mood and cognition.[186]

Probiotics also manufacture the B vitamins and vitamin K and improve digestive function. They are also important for immunity, as 70% of your immune system is in your gut, and we know they can alleviate[187] and prevent allergic diseases such as hay fever, food intolerances and eczema.

They improve detoxification and, through their role in improving digestion, they prevent food from sitting in the gut producing toxins. Both probiotics and prebiotics (which act a bit like fertiliser to promote the growth of the probiotics) also have anti-inflammatory effects.[188]

It's hard to imagine, but your digestive system contains 100,000 billion bacteria, weighing in at around a kilo (1kg) – or about two pounds (2lbs) – and, in with this mix, you need good levels of beneficial bacteria (probiotics) to help to keep control of the pathogenic bacteria, parasites and yeasts. There is a delicate bacterial balance to be had, and, unfortunately, our natural levels of probiotics fall as we get older. In addition, they are reduced in number, or even wiped out totally, if we use antibiotics, HRT, or the contraceptive pill – and stress also depletes them. This is important to know because your gut flora can help control whether you gain weight[189] and it can also influence your risk of becoming insulin resistant or developing type 2 diabetes.[190]

In fact, research has indicated that changing your levels of intestinal bacteria (without changing your diet) can influence whether you become overweight. In one fascinating study, scientists bred genetically identical mice and split them into two groups. One group was given the intestinal bacteria from an obese person and the other group was given the bacteria from that person's lean twin. The two groups of mice were kept on the same diet, eating the same amount as each other, but the mice that got the bacteria from the obese person became overweight and had more body fat than the mice given the bacteria from the lean person.[191]

In a similar human study, volunteers who were overweight and prediabetic were given the gut bacteria from slender volunteers with normal blood sugar. Within six weeks, the volunteers who had been prediabetic saw their insulin resistance improve. Their blood sugar stabilised, and they also lost weight.[192]

Another study, a few years later, showed similar results, but this study was longer and this time, after 18 weeks, the prediabetic volunteers returned to their prediabetic state and regained their weight.[193]

From this we can conclude that when your good bacteria are in balance, you are less susceptible to weight gain and insulin resistance, which in turn protects you from both prediabetes and type 2 diabetes. And these good bacteria have to be kept at good levels all the time, feeding them with a healthy diet containing fibre in addition to probiotic supplements. The broader the range of fibrous foods you eat, the more diverse your beneficial bacteria will become, and it is this diversity that is so vital for good health.

While eating diversely came naturally to our primitive ancestors, it's thought that these days 75% of the food in the world comes from only twelve plants and five animal species. And that, of the 300,000 edible plant species, we only eat about 200 of them.[194]

In fact, you may know people whose staple diet of meat and two veg revolves around the same two vegetables most days, without much variety at all.

To boost your intake of fibrous plant foods, think about different fruits, vegetables, wholegrains, legumes, nuts and seeds and be adventurous! Try foods that you haven't tried before.

It is much easier to do this now than when I started in the field of nutrition over 30 years ago. I remember walking into a health food shop, seeing the packets of dried beans on the shelves and not knowing what to do with them. It's great that you can now buy tins of ready cooked organic beans such as kidney beans which can easily be added to a casserole or stew. And you can further help your microbiome by eating the kinds of fermented foods that have been enjoyed by many traditional cultures for centuries. These include yoghurt, kimchi, sauerkraut, kefir and tempeh – all of which are easy to come by these days.

Do make the effort to diversify your diet with these foods, even if they are new to you and mean changing lifelong habits. Because it is clear that the usual Western diet – high in refined sugar and low in fibre – actively *reduces* the diversity of your gut bacteria. When researchers fed mice a low fibre diet for just four weeks, the mice had a 60% decrease in the different species within the gut.[195] They then switched the mice back to a high-fibre diet and half the microbial species returned to normal levels.

As I've already mentioned above, while *probiotics* are your beneficial bacteria, prebiotics are the foods that 'feed' these beneficial bacteria, and this group of foods includes onions, garlic, asparagus, legumes, oats and leeks. In a supplement, inulin and FOS (fructooligosaccharides) are the prebiotics you need to look for.

Prebiotics are just as important as probiotics for type 2 diabetes, as research has shown that they help control blood sugar levels and change the speed at which you would get a blood sugar spike from your food.[196]

If you need to take an antibiotic for an infection, take a probiotic throughout the course of antibiotics and for three months afterwards – but take the probiotic and antibiotic at different times of day. If you are on a medication that reduces your beneficial bacteria on a continual basis, such as HRT or the Pill, you might benefit from taking a probiotic all the time. However, I suggest you avoid probiotic drinks, which often have high amounts of added sugar, and instead choose a probiotic capsule containing at least 22 billion organisms – including both lactobacillus and bifidobacteria strains – that does not have to be refrigerated (it is freeze dried and only gets activated when you swallow it) and is, therefore, much more convenient, especially if you're travelling. Ideally also take a prebiotic like FOS (fructooligosaccharides), or a synbiotic, which is a combination of both probiotics and prebiotics in one supplement, so that they work synergistically in your digestive tract. The prebiotics will help the probiotics survive in your intestines. The probiotic I use in the clinic is NHP's Advanced Probiotic Support which is freeze dried and also contains a prebiotic and also gamma oryzanol to soothe digestive discomfort and glutamine to help with a leaky gut (see pages 152 and 230).

Avoid probiotics that contain maltodextrin. It is a synthetic polysaccharide, made up of glucose molecules, and is produced by the partial hydrolysis of starch (such as rice, corn or potato starch). Maltodextrin is quickly digested, because it is made up of glucose molecules, and it is absorbed as rapidly as glucose, and can affect your blood sugar levels. Research has also shown that it may suppress the anti-microbial defence mechanisms in your digestive system (it enabled Salmonella to survive in a study on mice) – and it could also make you more prone to inflammation.[197]

Could You Have A Leaky Gut?

Prebiotics are also important to help maintain the integrity of your intestinal barrier, and stop it from becoming 'leaky' – and it's thought that high blood sugar can increase the risk of having a leaky gut (intestinal permeability). Research has suggested that when bacteria leak through the gut they can trigger an inflammatory response that interferes with the effectiveness of insulin to control blood sugar effectively – and this contributes to insulin resistance.[198]

So, we have the scenario where a high sugar diet can cause a leaky gut, and a leaky gut can also lead to high blood sugar – which is why it is so important to not only stop your consumption of added sugar but also to 'feed' your gut bacteria with good levels of probiotic and prebiotics (in both food and supplements), in order to stop the vicious cycle.

Your gut should act as a barrier to prevent toxins, bacteria and large molecules escaping into your bloodstream. But when it becomes 'leaky' it loses the ability to act as a barrier and this increased permeability is associated with reacting inappropriately to some foods – and also increased susceptibility to autoimmune diseases, skin problems and inflammation in general. Having a gut that is too permeable allows food particles to escape through your gut wall and this sets up an immune reaction that makes you react negatively to certain foods. This is a food intolerance, though, and not the same as a true food allergy.

For information to help you diagnose a leaky gut, see Chapter 26.

Chapter 19

Herbal help

'It is wonderful that nature supplies us with herbs that can help prevent and treat type 2 diabetes.'

In your fight against insulin resistance, prediabetes and full-blown type 2 diabetes, you could easily find yourself on numerous medications as I have explained earlier in the book. On the other hand, you may be able to avoid drugs (and only if timely and appropriate) by adding the following herbs to your diet and supplement regime.

• Cinnamon (Ceylon)

Cinnamon has been shown to improve insulin sensitivity and also has a fat burning effect; and studies show that it can help reduce blood glucose levels and improve insulin resistance in those with type 2 diabetes.[199] A review of 16 studies on diabetes treatment found promising results for Ceylon cinnamon (Cinnamomum zeylanicum) in particular,[200] with the study's authors calling this cinnamon (which is native to Sri Lanka and parts of India) 'true' cinnamon. Not all cinnamon is created equal.

Cassia cinnamon, also known as Chinese cinnamon, is considered to be a lower quality and also contains high amounts of coumarin, which is potentially toxic and has an anti-coagulant effect. You need to be especially careful of cassia cinnamon if you are taking a blood thinner such as aspirin, heparin or warfarin. It is thought that even one or two teaspoons daily would be too much.

By contrast, Ceylon cinnamon contains such low levels of coumarin that it is often undetectable,[201] meaning it's safe to take even if you're on a blood-thinning medication.

It is also thought that many of cinnamon's bioactive compounds could help to block the protein in the brain (tau) from accumulating, which is characteristic of Alzheimer's. Research using Alzheimer's-diseased rats showed that 'true' cinnamon improves learning ability[202] and that it could have neuroprotective effects on the brain.

I consider cinnamon to be so important for type 2 diabetes that I recommend it as part of my supplement programme (see chapter 17), and it is included in NHP's Blood Sugar (Glucose) Support supplement.

Take: 200mg Ceylon cinnamon per day

• Garlic

Garlic has been used for centuries around the world, both as food and medicine, and it contains more than 400 compounds which have been found to be beneficial to blood pressure, cholesterol, immunity and fighting infection.

It is thought that many of these benefits are due to an active ingredient called allicin which is released when you chop or crush a raw clove of garlic. However, the benefits are weakened by cooking the garlic. The suggestion is to eat two to three raw garlic cloves a day (to avoid losing too many friends, chew parsley to offset the odour) – but it is probably easier to take a supplement. Indeed, garlic supplements have been found to reduce levels of fasting blood glucose and HbA1c in those with type 2 diabetes (and also to reduce total cholesterol and LDL ('bad') cholesterol).[203]

In one study, people with type 2 diabetes who were also taking metformin were given either a garlic supplement or a placebo (dummy pill). In those taking both metformin and the garlic, the combination was especially helpful in reducing fasting blood glucose and also decreasing total cholesterol, triglycerides and LDL cholesterol and improving HDL ('good') cholesterol[204] (and had more effect than the metformin with a dummy pill).

• Fenugreek

This is a herb that is often used in curries. The leaves can be used as a vegetable and the seeds are either used whole or powdered.

A study giving 10mg of soaked seeds in hot water to patients who had type 2 diabetes and were taking oral diabetes medication or insulin showed that taking the seeds significantly reduced fasting blood sugar and HbA1c. It took at least six months for the effect to be realised, so this is not a quick remedy. But it could help in the long term.[205] It is thought that the soluble fibre in the fenugreek seeds helps to lower blood sugar by slowing your digestion and absorption of carbohydrates.

• Ginger

This is a well-known herb that has been used around the world for many years and can be found in Indian, South Asian and Japanese dishes, and is also often drunk as a tea.

Ginger can help with nausea, joint pains and also digestive problems including indigestion, gas and bloating. But taking ginger as a supplement has been shown to help reduce fasting blood sugar and lower HbA1c[206] – and it can also help with weight loss. It's been shown to reduce waist-to-hip ratio and increase levels of healthy HDL cholesterol.[207]

• Turmeric

Turmeric has had a lot of press over the last few years as an anti-inflammatory herb that can help with arthritis. It is a root (rhizome) that is part of the ginger family (Zingiberaceae) and is native to India. You can add it to your cooking raw or as a powder or it can be taken in supplement form.

As with ginger, turmeric will taste fresher when used in its whole root form rather than as a powder, but for many people the powder is much more convenient. It is made by chopping and boiling the root and then drying it, so this will remove some important oils but many of its nutritional benefits are retained. It is thought that turmeric powder has a shelf life of up to three years if it's kept in a jar with a tight-fitting lid in a dark cupboard.

People in India have drunk turmeric with milk for many years as an Ayurvedic remedy. It is known as golden milk or Haldi Doodh. The practice has caught on in the West with people drinking turmeric lattes, sometimes made with milk or plant milk. Other spices such as ginger, cinnamon, black pepper and cardamom can also be added. I think if you are going to make your own then this can be a healthy choice for a drink and there are some organic powders already made up to use, but do read the labels as some will have added a sweetener.

The active component of turmeric, curcumin, is thought to be able to decrease blood sugar and can, therefore, play a role in diabetes prevention, as well as reducing many of the complications of diabetes.[208] Do be careful if you are on blood sugar lowering medication, in case curcumin lowers your blood sugar level too much.

• Gymnema Sylvestre

This is a plant that has been used for centuries in Pakistan and India, and traditionally has been used to help maintain healthy blood sugar. It seems to be able to make sweet foods taste less sweet so you can end up not wanting to eat so much of them. It is also called Gurmar which means sugar-destroyer.

It lowers your blood sugar and you would need to be careful if you are taking diabetic medication as it might cause your blood sugar to go too low. Its active ingredient is gymnemic acid which has antidiabetic and antiobesity properties.

Gymnemic acid delays glucose absorption in the blood and, because molecularly it is very close to glucose, it fills the glucose receptor locations on your taste buds preventing the activation of sugar molecules in the food so food tastes less sweet. As a result, your taste will alter, you'll become less sweet-toothed and you'll stop craving sweetness so much. The same mechanism happens in your digestive system and prevents the sugar molecules being absorbed so you have lower blood sugar levels.

• Bitter Melon (Karela)

This is another plant that has been used for centuries both as a food and medicine and it grows in tropical and subtropical climates. It has at least three active substances with antidiabetic properties, including charantin, vicine and an insulin-like compound called polypeptide-p. It helps to reduce blood sugar in people with type 2 diabetes[209] but not as efficiently as metformin.

• Ashwagandha

Ashwagandha is a plant that is grown in India, parts of Africa and the Middle East. It has been used medicinally for centuries and has anti-microbial, anti-inflammatory and antioxidant properties. Often used to help with anxiety, arthritis and sleep, it has also been shown to help lower blood sugar and reduce HbA1c[210] with results suggesting it could have a potential role in managing type 2 diabetes. Do be careful if you are on blood sugar lowering medication, in case the ashwagandha lowers your blood sugar level too much.

The Bottom Line

It is wonderful that nature supplies us with nutrients and herbs that can help prevent and treat type 2 diabetes. It is fine to use the vitamins, minerals, probiotics and omega 3 essential fats and cinnamon alongside any diabetes medication but always let your doctor know what you are taking – and do be cautious with the other herbs. If you are not on any diabetic medication then they are worth trying but, as I've shown, they could lower your blood sugar too much – so you would need to be monitored if you are already taking medication that's doing the same thing.

Chapter 20

What do you eat
and *when* do you eat it?

"Research supports a 12:12 pattern of eating, with a 12 hour overnight fast."

We have always known that WHAT you eat is important for preventing and treating type 2 diabetes as well as for your general health. But in the last few years it has become clear that WHEN you eat also really matters.

We all now know the term 'intermittent fasting' and you may already have tried one of the variations of this popular way to lose weight and reduce blood glucose and cholesterol.

One of the first of these fasting regimes was the 5:2 diet, which requires you to fast on two days a week, but eat normally on the remaining five. However, it has never been clear whether the two days of fasting work better when they are consecutive (for example, every Tuesday and Wednesday) or when they are broken up (say, Tuesday and Friday) and there has also been debate about whether the fasting days should involve a complete fast – with nothing except water – or the popular alternative of 600 calories for men and 500 calories for women.

And, if you follow the 5:2 fast with restricted calories, there is no definite research yet to say whether it is better to have all the calories in one meal or spread out throughout the day.

Other regimes suggest alternate day fasting, where you are fasting every other day of the week.

There is also the 16:8 version, where you only eat within an eight-hour period each day (for example between 10am and 6pm) but fast the rest of the time.

No matter which pattern you are following, the suggestion curiously seems to be that you can eat anything you like, and however much you want, during the non-fasting hours. There is no counting of calories and there are no recommendations about which foods to eat or avoid.

Research has suggested that intermittent fasting could help reduce the risk of both prediabetes and type 2 diabetes.[211] And it can lower HbA1c in people with type 2 diabetes, as well as those following a calorie restricted diet.[212]

It is thought that intermittent fasting might be easier to follow for some people than restricting calories. But research in 2021 showed that those who fasted on alternate days lost fewer pounds than those who were eating the same number of calories but not fasting. Those who weren't fasting lost just over four pounds (1.8kg) over the three weeks of the trial with all the weight being lost as fat. But the individuals following the alternative day fasting lost three and a half pounds (1.6kg) but the weight lost was half fat and half muscle. This matters a lot as the type of weight lost is crucial! You don't want to lose muscle, as it is metabolically active and helps you to burn fat even when you are resting.[213]

I also don't think this way of eating is suitable for everyone. If you are pregnant, breastfeeding, under 18, or have a history of an eating disorder then you shouldn't follow this regime – and nor is it good for anyone who is very stressed or suffering from chronic fatigue. Your body experiences fasting as a form of stress, because it perceives that there is a shortage of food, which, in primitive terms, is a life or death survival issue. So, if you are already stressed or fatigued you cannot afford to add another stress – lack of food – to your body.

If you do a lot of exercise or are training for an event then you would also need to think carefully about this kind of diet.

Also, it seems that this way of eating is not suitable for women, as one study found that blood sugar control actually got worse in women after doing intermittent fasting for three weeks.[214] And we also already know that when women restrict their calories, there can be repercussions for their menstrual cycle – and, as is well known, women who lose too much weight can see their cycles can stop completely.

Studies on female rats have shown that three to six months of intermittent fasting actually shrinks the ovaries and causes irregular menstrual cycles.[215]

Feast Or Famine?

For many years, the popular theory has been that dietary restriction helps us live longer – that it is a survival mechanism to conserve energy when food is scarce, during a famine for example, and that when food availability is low the body goes into maintaining and repairing itself and benefits long term survival.

But interesting research on fruit flies, which are often used as a 'stand-in' for humans, has shown that switching back to a plentiful diet after cutting consumption causes the female flies to lay fewer eggs and die prematurely.[216] The researchers are clear to point out that fruit flies are not us, but they wonder if switching from restriction to normal eating on a regular basis within short periods of time could have negative health consequences.

Normally, when fruit flies' diets are restricted their risk of death drops significantly but if they eat a rich diet after restriction it seems to cause an 'overshoot' effect and the flies have a very high mortality rate. It is possible that sudden changes in diet are harmful, and it is consistency that our bodies need rather than 'all or nothing'.

This is clear from research into yo-yo dieting – where weight is lost and then regained, and usually involves trying different and often extreme diets over time – which more than doubles your risk of an early death and increases your risks of type 2 diabetes, high cholesterol, high blood pressure, heart attack and stroke.[217]

As mentioned above, the 16:8 diet is one of those regimes that tells you *when* to eat – i.e., within an eight-hour window of time – yet gives no advice about *what* to eat within that timeframe. Basically, someone could be living on fast food and takeaways during those eight hours, which is obviously not going to be a good idea by any stretch of the imagination!

You will benefit far more from knowing what to eat – and sticking to the healthy eating advice I'm setting out in this book – and combining this knowledge with some sense of timing, so you take full advantage of your circadian rhythm.

Eat Little And Often

Do any of these symptoms sound familiar? Run through the following checklist and tick off the ones that you experience on a regular basis:

- Irritability
- Aggressive outbursts
- Nervousness, fears and anxiety
- Depression
- Crying spells
- Dizziness
- Confusion, forgetfulness, inability to concentrate
- Fatigue
- Insomnia
- Headaches
- Palpitations
- Muscle cramps
- Excess sweating
- Digestive problems
- Allergies
- Lack of sex drive

These are all symptoms of low blood sugar (hypoglycaemia) caused by your blood sugar rising too high and then crashing back down. To keep your blood sugar balanced and to avoid the dips (low blood sugar, hypoglycaemia) that will send you racing off to get a quick fix with a chocolate bar or a packet of biscuits, make sure that you are eating little and often.

My recommendation is to have a good breakfast, lunch and dinner and also to include a mid-morning and a mid-afternoon snack. Don't go longer than three hours without eating (this is especially vital for women) or your blood sugar levels will drop too low and your body will give you a craving for something sweet to rectify the drop quickly.

If you miss breakfast, you are setting yourself up to fail because by 11am you will be craving a coffee and a Danish because your blood sugar will have dropped so low. Remember that breakfast means 'breaking the fast'. You have not eaten since dinner the night before and that first meal of the day is the one that *breaks the fast*. Of course, it needs to be a good breakfast. If you opt for a sugary breakfast cereal, this will give a quick rise in blood sugar followed by a drop soon afterwards, giving you the feeling that you need another quick fix to keep you going and so it goes on.

Breakfast can give you the biggest insulin spike of the day if you are starting the day with cereal. Interestingly, research has shown that if people with well managed type 2 diabetes switch their breakfast from cereal (high carb) to omelette (low carb, high fat), they don't get an immediate blood sugar spike after breakfast, have lowered glucose levels in general, and maintain their blood sugar stability over the next 24 hours. The participants of this study also had reduced cravings for sweet things when they had an omelette for breakfast rather than cereal.[218]

Follow A 12:12 Pattern Of Eating

The 16:8 diet is difficult to do, and I would suggest you don't follow this pattern of eating if you have type 2 diabetes.

The best way to time your food is to follow the 12:12 pattern of eating (and the research is really good on this regime). This is called time-restricted eating and is a form of intermittent fasting but much more practical and convenient than starving yourself on a number of days a week. You could have your breakfast at 7am and dinner at 7pm and then you are basically fasting overnight.

You should aim to leave at least two to three hours from your last meal before you go to bed. So, if dinner is at 7pm then you would go to bed around 10 or 11pm. This is so important because the timing of your evening meal affects your metabolism and glucose control. Researchers at Johns Hopkins Medicine studied 20 healthy volunteers by giving them a meal at a traditional hour (6pm) or the same meal at a later time of the day (10pm). All went to bed at 11pm. When the volunteers had the late meal, they burnt 10% less fat overnight than when they stopped eating three hours before they went to bed.[219] And the late meal caused 18% higher levels of glucose than the same meal eaten at 6pm. Also, those who had the late meal had higher glucose and insulin levels two hours after eating breakfast.

The researchers found that when people ate later, they had higher spikes in blood sugar, slower fat breakdown and even increases in the stress hormone cortisol, believed to be a factor in promoting weight gain. When they looked more closely at different responses to the late meal, they found that people who normally went to bed early — so-called "early birds" — experienced an even bigger impact from eating late.

As the researchers said, '**What time you eat** could be just as important as **what you eat** when it comes to metabolic health' and 'when people eat identical meals at two different times, their bodies apparently process those calories differently. How an individual responds depends on their particular biorhythms and sleep behaviors'.[220]

Interesting recent research from Italy, presented at the European Congress on Obesity in 2020, analysed a group of obese people and looked at the time they woke in the morning and the time they went to bed. The night owls who went to bed later were six times more likely to develop type 2 diabetes (and also four times more likely to have heart disease) than the morning larks (the early risers).

We all have different chronotypes – that is, the time we prefer to get up and the time we go to bed, and is the basic difference between night owls and morning larks. And it is known that if you are an evening chronotype – a night owl who prefers to stay up later – you have a higher risk of obesity, metabolic syndrome and insulin resistance.[221] And it is also thought that being an evening chronotype might predispose you to different behaviours such as eating foods that are higher in fat, drinking more alcohol, eating in places other than the kitchen or dining room (maybe in bed), eating straight out of a packet, stress related (comfort) eating and even taking less physical activity.[222] The most powerful take-home message from this research is that this is not a genetic risk but a behaviour that is modifiable. So, by changing your pattern of activities, you can take control of the situation and either prevent type 2 diabetes or help to treat it. And it is now becoming clear that what you eat at different times of the day can have different effects on your weight, even if you are eating exactly the same food with the same amount of calories. One example is that when you eat more in the morning than in the evening, you are less likely to be overweight or obese.[223]

A really interesting study took a group of overweight and obese women and split them into two groups. Both groups ate 1400 calories a day for 12 weeks. But WHEN they ate those calories differed.

The 'breakfast' group:

Breakfast   700 calories

Lunch   500 calories

Dinner   200 calories

The 'dinner' group:

Breakfast   200 calories

Lunch   500 calories

Dinner   700 calories

Lunch stayed the same in both groups, the only difference was switching round breakfast and dinner.

The group that had higher calories for breakfast had greater weight loss and lost more inches from their waist. Their fasting glucose and insulin levels decreased significantly more than those in the 'dinner' group. Triglycerides decreased by 33.6% in the 'breakfast group', but increased by 14.6% in the 'dinner' group. And the 'breakfast' group also felt more satisfied with their food.[224]

Breakfast is important, because it is 'breaking the fast', and if you skip breakfast just one day a week it can increase your risk of developing type 2 diabetes by six per cent. Miss it four to five days a week increases the risk to 55%.[225] And you also have a 55% higher risk of becoming overweight or obese.

This 12:12 pattern of eating can help with weight management, improving sleep and reducing the risk of cardiovascular disease.[226] Overweight people asked to eat only during a maximum of a 12-hour window for 16 weeks lost weight, had more energy, and slept better – and these benefits lasted for a year.[227]

Remember: you are insulin sensitive at the beginning of the day and you become more insulin resistant as the day goes on.[228] Therefore, the more you eat earlier in the day, the better your body can manage it. This old saying is still relevant but harder with our daily working habits: ***Breakfast like a king, lunch like a prince, and dinner like a pauper***!

As my recommendation is to combine both the 12:12 eating pattern and the 'little and often' regime, a good daily schedule would be:

7am breakfast

10am snack

1pm lunch

4pm snack

7pm dinner

You have no longer than three hours between food during the day, which keeps your blood sugar stable, and you will have about three hours or more between dinner and going to bed, and effectively a 12 hour fast overnight between 7am and 7pm.

Autophagy

You have a wonderful process in your body called autophagy and it is a housekeeping system that clears out dead cells and pathogens and enables newer, healthier cells to be regenerated.

It has been talked about a lot recently in terms of anti-ageing and also cancer prevention. All cancers start with abnormal cells and your body should recognise these cells as abnormal and remove them. And the thinking is that autophagy may lower the risk of cancer and also be good for your brain function and risk of Alzheimer's.[229]

Fasting seems to be the easiest way to trigger autophagy, hence all the interest in intermittent fasting. Following a keto diet also can trigger autophagy.

You can trigger the process of autophagy by following the 12:12 pattern of eating mentioned on page 162 and it means you don't have to fast during the day. You can also trigger autophagy by leaving three hours between your last meal of the day and going to bed, and then not eating for 12 hours. This is far easier to achieve than starving yourself for two or more days a week. It just means you have your evening meal at 8pm, go to bed at 11pm and then have breakfast at 8am.

Portion Size

Of course, the quality of your food is really important and the choices you make are key to preventing and reversing type 2 diabetes. But we must also think about the quantity too. Losing weight is really important to controlling type 2 diabetes so the amount you eat is crucial. Remember that your brain takes 20 minutes to register that you are full and satisfied so the slower you eat the less you will eat naturally: automatic portion control.

Below Are The Correct Serving Sizes For Different Foods:

Food	Serving Size	Use as size guide
Brown rice (cooked)	½ cup	Small muffin case
100% wholegrain bread	1 slice	
Potato (boiled or steamed)	1 small unit	Computer mouse/bar of soap
Potato (mashed)	½ cup	Small muffin case
Wholegrain pasta (cooked)	1 cup	1 cup
Dry cereal/porridge	30g	Small white wine glass
Cheese	45g	3 – 4 dice/domino
Natural yoghurt	125ml	Small tub
Nut butter	3 tsp	
Animal protein e.g. fish	150g	Palm of hand/deck of cards
Nuts	Small handful	
Mayonnaise	1-2 tsp	
Vinaigrette	1 tbsp	
Vegetables	½ - 1 cup	Tennis ball
Fruit – apple/pear/orange	1 small unit	
Berries	1 cup	
Dried fruit	1½ tbsp	
Stewed fruit	⅓ cup	

I have left in some foods that you are best avoiding, e.g. potatoes, just in case you have them served to you when you're out socially and it would be awkward to avoid them. These are the maximum amounts you should eat and if more have been put on your plate then you should leave them.

Use Smaller Plates

Research shows that the larger our plates, the more food we put on them, and the more we eat – regardless of our appetite![230] This is really important when you are faced with a buffet. Pick up a side plate rather than the large dinner plate as it is very easy to pile a lot of food onto the plate and harder when the plate is smaller.

Also, although you may have been told this as a child, you do not have to finish everything on your plate. Turn the old habit around. Each time you eat, try to make a habit of leaving something on your plate and over time you will realise that you are eating less without even thinking about it.

Be A Mindful Eater

Also called conscious eating, *mindful eating* is about being aware while you are eating. This is important because studies show you can eat up to 70% more than you realise if you're distracted by the TV. Even eating lunch in front of your computer makes you less likely to remember what you have eaten and more likely to feel hungry later. In one study, computer users ate twice as many biscuits half an hour after lunch at their desk than the non-computer users![231]

So, when you eat, take time to sit down and eat calmly. Many of my patients tell me they eat standing up (particularly breakfast), grabbing mouthfuls of something, while trying to get ready. Put your cutlery down between mouthfuls and enjoy every bite. Eat in a relaxed way, chew your food well and think of the food as the nourishment and fuel that is going to get you through the day.

Don't Skip Meals

Skipping meals can increase your risk of type 2 diabetes and also high blood pressure, high cholesterol and heart disease. Research from Sweden's Karolinska Institute revealed that irregular eating has damaging effects, even if your diet is fairly healthy. The team studied 3,607 women and men aged 60 and showed that skipping meals increases the risk of insulin resistance by up to 60%.[232] Your body needs consistency, so make sure you have regularity with the timing of your meals and don't skip them.

Get to understand your hunger cues, as it may be easy to override them because you don't realise you are hungry, or you think you don't have time to eat. You might not have a growling stomach that tells you it is time to eat. You might start to feel light-headed or dizzy, or feel your energy has dropped – this kind of slump is very common around 3 or 4pm in the afternoon. Or you might start to get shaky or irritable. All of these are signalling that your blood sugar is dropping and you need to eat.

Don't Eat On The Run

As well as not skipping meals, don't eat on the run. Many workers nowadays do not take a full lunch hour and will often skip lunch. Often people worry that by taking time out to eat they will be giving their bosses a negative impression.

But if you eat on the run, grabbing a sandwich at lunchtime whilst still working at your desk, or rushing off to meet someone and eating the sandwich on the way, you will not digest your food properly. You won't absorb adequately the goodness from that food and will end up feeling bloated and uncomfortable. You may also get loose bowel motions or even diarrhoea, as stress hormones relax the rectum muscles.

Change How You Think About Food

A lot of patients talk to me about food being 'good' or 'bad', or they say about themselves that they have been 'really good with the food this week'. When food is labelled like this there can be a lot of guilt around 'being bad' or eating 'bad' foods.

It is better to think of your food as 'healthy' or 'unhealthy' and use those labels to help you choose those foods that are going to nourish you back into good health and reverse type 2 diabetes.

And think of food as the fuel you put into your body to give yourself the energy to do the things you want to do. As an analogy, if you put poor quality fuel into a high-performance car it may run for a while but eventually it will become less efficient, the engine will deteriorate, and it will get age faster. It is exactly the same with your body. You need top grade fuel to run on all four cylinders. Providing your body with nourishing foods will help to keep you healthy, slow down the ageing process, and prevent and treat type 2 diabetes and many other degenerative diseases such as heart disease, cancer and Alzheimer's.

Have Soup Before A Meal

If you have soup before a meal you should end up eating fewer calories during the meal because soup stops the cells in the stomach producing your hunger hormone ghrelin and, hence, turns off your appetite.

Studies show the body registers greater satisfaction when food is liquidised, and soup also moves out of the stomach more gradually than a solid meal would, leaving you feeling more satisfied for longer.

Make Sure You Are Drinking Enough Water

I've discussed the importance of drinking enough water in Chapter 16. Do take this seriously. Allowing yourself to become dehydrated can cause high blood sugar.

Make Friends With Apple Cider Vinegar

It is thought that apple cider vinegar drunk just before meals can help reduce the blood sugar rise that follows the meal. It is thought that the apple cider vinegar slows down the conversion of carbohydrates into sugar entering the bloodstream. One meta-analysis which looked at six studies on 317 participants found that apple cider vinegar reduced fasting blood glucose and HbA1c.[233] There was also a reduction in total cholesterol and LDL ('bad' cholesterol).

I would suggest buying organic raw apple cider vinegar and mixing about one teaspoon into water as drinking it neat can be irritating to your stomach.

Some Other Tips:

- Fill half your plate at lunch and dinner with vegetables.

- Don't go back for seconds or keep dishes of food on the table.

- There's no need to finish the plate!

- Remember to eat slowly, chew properly and enjoy your food.

- Are you really hungry – or dehydrated? Lack of water can make you think you are hungry for food, leading to overeating and weight gain.

- Tidy up your leftovers. Put everything away in portion size containers as soon as you have served.

- When eating prepared food:
  – Check label for portion size.
  – Always take food out of the container and put on a plate.
  – Don't eat in front of the TV.

- When eating out:
  – Get rid of the breadbasket or just have one small piece.
  – Order a soup and a starter or two starters.
  – Have extra vegetables instead of potatoes / pasta / rice / bread.
  – Share your food!

- Drink from a smaller wine or beer glass.

- Take a long-term view. There will be times when you slip up and overeat or pick less healthy foods. Healthy eating is a long-term strategy and the occasional slip won't make any difference in the long run. Think of the 80:20 rule. If you overdo it one day, eat less the following day to redress the balance.

• **Know What To Eat**

Include:

Unrefined complex carbohydrates like brown rice, whole wheat, oats, wild rice, oatmeal, millet, barley.

Quinoa – it cooks up like rice so can be used like a starchy carbohydrate, but it is actually a seed and high in protein and rich in vitamins and minerals.

Fruit (always whole, not juiced) – especially apples, berries, cherries, kiwi fruit, oranges, peaches, grapefruit, pears, plums, strawberries.

Non-starchy vegetables as listed on page 104.

Nuts.

Seeds.

Protein – good quality like fish, especially oily fish (salmon, herring, tuna) and eggs.

Dairy – especially yoghurt and ideally organic.

Legumes – lentils, aduki beans, chickpeas (including humus), kidney beans, pinto beans, soya beans (tofu).

Avoid:

Anything containing sugar, like pastries, cakes, sweets and including drinks.

Refined carbohydrates like white bread, white rice, white pasta.

Starchy vegetables – eat in moderation, see page 103.

Fruit flavoured yoghurts and probiotic drinks.

Dried fruit – keep to a minimum and only have with a protein like nuts and seeds.

Fruit juice.

Any foods containing trans fats – look for the words 'hydrogenated vegetable oil' on the label.

Any foods or drinks containing artificial sweeteners.

The Bottom Line

You want to get to a situation where your way of eating becomes a way of life. This is not a diet that you follow for a short while and then abandon and go back to your former eating patterns that caused the type 2 diabetes in the first place.

The idea is that you embrace a whole new concept of nourishing yourself that is full of variety and taste. By eliminating foods that are not good for you and concentrating on foods that are healthy, you will find this becomes a way of life that is easy to follow – I promise you won't feel deprived.

There may be occasions when it is not possible to follow the guidelines exactly, perhaps when you are being entertained by others. So long as you have a foundation of eating well, then the odd deviation will not matter. Remember the 80/20 rule – and shrug aside the 'naughty' 20% and focus on making the vast majority of your food health-giving and kind to your body. Above all, food is to be enjoyed. Eating is a time for sharing and socialising. There is nothing more demoralising than turning down invites to eat with friends because you can't share their food.

Chapter 21

Carbs v ketones

"Only follow a keto diet if your doctor has recommended it and you are being monitored – especially if you already have type 2 diabetes and are on medication."

A low fat diet used to be considered the best way to lose weight. The reverse of this is the ketogenic diet. But is it really as useful a tool as some suggest? And what can it do for you if you have type 2 diabetes or are at risk of it?

The ketogenic diet is basically one that is high in fat (75% of your calories) and lower in carbohydrates (five to 10%) with moderate amounts of protein. Your body normally gets energy from the carbohydrates that you eat, but because the carbohydrate content is very low in this diet, it shifts its energy source to use fat for fuel – and this produces ketones as the fats in your liver are broken down. Inducing 'nutritional ketosis' is the aim of the ketogenic diet. Restricting carbohydrates causes your body to produce more ketones to help with weight loss – and initial weight loss can appear to be good – up to six kg (one stone) in the first week – but a large part of this can be water loss, not fat.

What's happening is that, when your body is starved of carbohydrate, it looks for energy from your glycogen stores; and because four grams (0.14oz) of water cling to every single gram of glycogen, it is possible to lose a lot of weight very quickly – but this is often called losing 'water weight'. When your glycogen stores are depleted your body starts to burn the fat. This happens very slowly so it seems that the diet has stopped working. But it can take a few weeks for your body to adapt to using ketones for energy instead of carbohydrates, so you would need to be patient with this diet.

A ketogenic style of diet has been scientifically proven to help people with epilepsy to reduce the number of seizures and has been used since the 1920s, for this purpose. (When someone is having a seizure, neurons fire inappropriately and brain cells release more excitatory neurotransmitters like glutamate. It is thought that the ketogenic diet reduces the amount of glutamate in the brain and reduces the excitability that triggers the seizures.) It is only fairly recently that it has become popular and mentioned in the media as another 'fad' weight loss diet. But a large new study has suggested that, in the long term, it can actually increase the risk of a number of long-term, life-threatening illnesses including heart disease, cancer, Alzheimer's, and yes… diabetes! The study also showed, that for some people, it will raise LDL ('bad' cholesterol) and increase the likelihood of kidney problems (which can be a problem with type 2 diabetes anyway).[234]

Despite this study showing that it can increase the risk of type 2 diabetes, other research has looked at whether a ketogenic diet could actually prevent it. It doesn't seem to – except where the emphasis has been on vegetable rather than animal protein, in which case there was an 18% lower risk[235] of developing the disease and those who already had diabetes saw significant improvements to their blood sugar and HbA1c, as well as to the gut bacteria that are responsible for insulin sensitivity and lower levels of inflammation.[236]

As a further potential aid to type 2, the diet has been shown to be more successful than a low-fat diet for both weight loss and reducing HbA1c.[237] And it can decrease appetite, promote weight loos and decrease HbA1c in the short term. **But – and this is a big but – the research is suggesting that the reductions in HbA1c wane after a few months and that this type of diet is ultimately no more effective than any other**.[238]

A ketogenic diet is not an easy one to follow, and it can cause 'keto flu' where the change from how your body gets its energy source can give you side-effects such fatigue, headaches, muscle aches and nausea. You can also experience bad breath (a fruity odour of acetone – the same chemical as in nail polish remover), poorer concentration, mood swings, cravings for carbohydrate-rich foods and a bad memory.

You may also find that you get constipated from this way of eating because fibre-rich carbohydrates are missing – but sometimes people get diarrhoea because the higher fat content is causing the liver to release more bile, and this acts as a laxative.

And the other major concern of following this type of diet is on your gut microbiome. We know that your beneficial bacteria are important for your general health, weight loss and also the risk of developing type 2 diabetes (see Chapter 18) and yet it is thought that the ketogenic diet may have a negative effect on your gut microbes because of the lack of fibre that the beneficial bacteria 'feed' on (it is the same concern around someone staying on the FODMAP diet for too long). And because it is not an easy diet to stick with, if you veer off the diet, the weight will pile back on quickly.

I would suggest that you only follow a keto diet if your doctor has recommended it and you are being monitored – especially if you already have type 2 diabetes and are on medication.

In the recent words of researchers: *'current evidence suggests that for most individuals, the risks of such diets outweigh the benefits.'*[239]

Diabetic Ketoacidosis (DKA)

You might have heard about this problem and seen the connection with the word 'keto' and wondered how it differs from nutritional ketosis, which is the aim of the ketogenic diet.

Whereas with nutritional ketosis, your body can regulate the ketones so that they do not get too high, DKA is a potentially life-threatening condition and occurs in those with type 1 diabetes who have not used enough insulin. The ketone levels rise to about 10 times higher than those found in nutritional ketosis and, in this situation, the body has too much glucose in the blood but not enough insulin to move the glucose (sugar) out of the blood into the cells to use for energy. The person's body then thinks it is starving and breaks down fats and proteins too quickly. This leads to high levels of ketones *and* blood sugar, and makes the blood too acidic (a condition called acidosis), which can change how certain organs in your body function, notably your liver and kidneys.

With ketosis there will be high levels of ketones in the blood or urine but not high enough to cause acidosis. Ketones can be measured with a urine dipstick. These identify when you have reached nutritional ketosis and the tables below shows the different levels.

Urine Ketone Levels	<0.5 mmol/L	>0.5 mmol/L	0.5-3 mmol/L
What Do My Ketone Levels Mean?	Normal to low	Beginning ketosis	Nutritional ketosis (ideal for purposeful ketosis)

Urine Ketone Levels	>3–5 mmol/L	>5 mmol/L	>10 mmol/LU
What Do My Ketone Levels Mean?	Starvation ketosis	High risk for ketoacidosis (if blood sugar is greater than 250 mg/dL, call your doctor)	DKA (seek medical attention immediately)

Tables from https://www.healthline.com/health/ketosis-vs-ketoacidosis#diagnosis

<hr>

Chapter 22

Meal planners

"Please, just tell me what to eat!"

When you are making changes to your diet, it helps to know why you are making those changes, *how* to make healthier choices and what is best to eat. It can be complex and confusing, and my own patients frequently say, 'please, just tell me what to eat!'

I hope the meal planners in this chapter will help you move forward with confidence.

Feel free to mix and match your meals. You will have some favourites that you don't mind repeating, and you may have dietary preferences such as oat milk instead of dairy. I would suggest buying organic produce (including organic dairy milk) wherever possible and, if you're drinking a plant 'milk', do read the ingredients as some can contain added sugar.

I haven't included any meat or poultry and that is a personal choice from me in that I have excluded those for the last 30 or so years. Eat them if you want to, but make sure you get the best quality you can and, again, preferably organic. But try to prioritise plant-based choices.

These meal plans assume that you will probably only be cooking for others once a day and able to choose your own food for breakfast and lunch. If you are at home during the week, your food choices will be easier to make, but many of us are at work during the day and that can make it harder to stick to healthy choices, so I've included advice about what to eat in restaurants.

Most of us do not have much time for preparing meals except when we are expecting guests, so meals on a day-to-day basis need to be quick and easy to prepare and yet healthy and nutritious. Therefore, the recipes I have given for the meal plans are mainly quick and simple – with just a few being more involved, for when you have more time. They can all be adapted to suit how much time you have and what you have available in your store cupboard.

Remember: if the foundations of what you eat in your day-to-day work and home life are healthy, it's not a disaster if you sometimes include less healthy foods when you eat out (it's that 80:20 rule).

As well as the meal plans, I have also included recipes that are mentioned in these plans plus desserts and sauces and these can be downloaded at: www.marilynglenville.com/diabetes-recipes

WEEK 1	Monday	Tuesday	Wednesday	Thursday	Friday	Saturday	Sunday
Breakfast	Porridge made with water + berries, ground mixed seeds and a spoon of natural yoghurt	1 slice wholemeal or rye toast + 1 poached or boiled egg	Natural probiotic yoghurt with sugar-free muesli, berries, chopped nuts	Porridge with fruit compote and milk, berries and mixed seeds (recipe 3)	Muesli with oat milk, berries and mixed seeds (recipe 4)	1 slice wholemeal or rye toast with nut butter	Scrambled eggs and tomatoes or mushrooms on 1 slice rye toast
Mid-morning snack	2 oatcakes with thin spread hummus	Pear and small handful mixed nuts	2 oatcakes with thin spread hummus	1 wholegrain cracker with cottage cheese and cucumber	Small pot natural probiotic yoghurt with flaked almonds	1 wholegrain cracker with cottage cheese and cucumber	Pear and small handful mixed nuts
Lunch	Carrot & chickpea soup	Tinned salmon mashed with probiotic yoghurt + salad	Hardboiled egg with avocado and mixed salad	Healthy salmon burger with mixed salad (recipe 6)	Vegetable and lentil soup (recipe 1)	Smoked or tinned mackerel and salad with watercress, spinach, cucumber and rocket	Frittata made with roasted butternut squash, spinach and herbs with green salad (recipe 2)
Mid-afternoon snack	Apple and 7 almonds	Vegetable sticks with 1/3 tub hummus	Small handful mixed nuts	Small tub natural probiotic yoghurt with handful berries	Orange and 5 brazil nuts	Small handful mixed nuts	Vegetable sticks with 1/3 tub hummus
Dinner	Asian salmon with steamed vegetables (recipe 23)	Quick tofu casserole with mixed vegetables (recipe 5)	Healthy salmon burger with salad of lettuce, grated carrot, cucumber, scallion, tomato (recipe 6)	Vegetable and prawn stir fry (recipe 13)	Grilled mackerel with crunchy salad	Frittata made with roasted butternut squash, spinach and herbs with green salad	Roast vegetable ratatouille with cod and butterbeans (recipe 7)

WEEK 2	Monday	Tuesday	Wednesday	Thursday	Friday	Saturday	Sunday
Breakfast	2 egg omelette with spinach, 1/2 red pepper and mushroom	Small portion of porridge made with water, natural probiotic yoghurt + handful blueberries	Boiled egg with one slice of wholegrain toast + apple	Small portion of porridge made with water, frozen berries and natural probiotic yoghurt	Berries with natural probiotic yoghurt and small handful flaked almonds or other nuts	Muesli (week 1 recipe) with natural probiotic yoghurt and grated pear / apple	Fresh fruit salad with natural probiotic yoghurt and flaked almonds
Mid-morning snack	2 sticks celery dipped in 1/4 tub cottage cheese	1 apple and 7 almonds	2 oatcakes with thin spread hummus	1 pear and small handful mixed seeds	1 wholegrain cracker with thin spread nut butter	2 oatcakes with thin spread hummus	Vegetable sticks and 1/3 tub hummus
Lunch	Leek and pea soup, wholegrain or rye bread (recipe 9)	Tandoori salmon salad with lettuce, scallion, cucumber, 1/2 avocado	Leek and pea soup, wholegrain or rye bread	Salad niçoise with tuna, lettuce, cucumber, spring onion, egg and tomato	Tinned salmon mashed with probiotic yoghurt + salad	Smoked salmon and avocado on rye bread smeared with horseradish sauce, mixed salad	Frittata with spinach, tomatoes and goat's cheese and side salad
Mid-afternoon snack	6 Brazil nuts + plum	2 oatcakes with cottage cheese	Small tub natural yoghurt with handful berries	Cucumber and pepper dipped in 1/3 tub hummus	1 satsuma and 7 walnut halves	Small tub natural yoghurt with handful berries	1 wholegrain cracker with cottage cheese
Dinner	Tandoori salmon with steamed vegetables (recipe 8)	Spanish fish stew with green beans (recipe 11)	Vegetable and prawn stir fry (recipe 13)	Ratatouille with butterbeans and feta (recipe 12)	Thai prawn curry	Frittata with spinach, tomatoes and goat's cheese and side salad (recipe 10)	Grilled fish fillet with 1 tsp pesto and steamed vegetables

WEEK 3	Monday	Tuesday	Wednesday	Thursday	Friday	Saturday	Sunday
Breakfast	Homemade no added sugar muesli with grated apple or pear + coconut milk (recipe 3)	Natural probiotic yoghurt with fresh fruit salad topped with ground seeds	1 slice wholemeal or rye toast, 1 poached egg, grilled tomatoes	Porridge with fruit compote and – tomatoes, feta cheese and olives with 1 slice rye bread	Greek breakfast	Grilled mushrooms and tomatoes and hummus on ½ a wholegrain bagel/rye bread	Berries with natural probiotic yoghurt and small handful flaked almonds of other nuts
Mid-morning snack	2 oatcakes with guacamole and cucumber	Small handful mixed nuts	Nectarine and 6 walnuts	1 rye cracker with edamame bean dip (recipe 14)	Apple and 4 Brazil nuts	2 wholegrain rice cakes with edamame dip (recipe 14)	Pear and 7 almonds
Lunch	Smoked salmon and avocado on rye bread smeared with horseradish sauce and green salad	Fritata with salad	Vegetable and Lentil Soup (recipe 1)	Wholemeal pitta stuffed with tinned mackerel fillets, spinach, tomatoes and cucumber	Vegetable and Lentil Soup (recipe 1) / large salad with mixed beans, spring onions, cucumber, mixed leaves, avocado	Salad of beans, dried cranberries, cucumber, radish and parsley	Baked sweet potato with a filling of tuna + sweetcorn mixed with a little natural yoghurt
Mid-afternoon snack	Tub natural probiotic yoghurt, berries and ground linseeds	Vegetable sticks with guacamole	Small tub probiotic yoghurt with berries	Mug minestrone soup	2 oatcakes with edamame bean dip (recipe 14)	1 orange and small handful sunflower seeds	2 wholegrain rice cakes with nut butter
Dinner	Leek, pea and bean frittata with mixed salad	Vegetable chili (recipe 15)	Healthy salmon burger (recipe 6)	Omelette with spinach, mushrooms and goat's cheese	Vegetable and prawn stir fry	Cod spread with 2 tsp pesto and baked, served with steamed vegetables	Frittata made with roasted butternut squash, spinach and herbs with green salad (recipe 10)

WEEK 4	Monday	Tuesday	Wednesday	Thursday	Friday	Saturday	Sunday
Breakfast	Muesli with berries, cinnamon, natural probiotic yoghurt, ground seeds	Natural probiotic yoghurt with fresh fruit salad topped with ground seeds	1 slice wholemeal or rye toast + 1 poached egg with grilled tomatoes	Slice of wholemeal or rye bread with peanut butter and 1/2 banana / 1 apple	Porridge with grated apple, cinnamon and flaked almonds	2 scrambled eggs and grilled mushrooms and tomatoes	Fruit salad with natural probiotic yoghurt and sprinkled with 2 tbsp muesli
Mid-morning snack	1 rye cracker with mackerel pate (recipe 16) and cucumber	2 oatcakes with hummus	1 rye cracker with mackerel pate + celery or tomato	2 oatcakes with hummus	Pear and sunflower seeds	Rye cracker, 1/2 banana, peanut butter	Celery sticks filled with cottage cheese, sprinkled with sunflower seeds
Lunch	Tomato and lentil soup (recipe 17) + slice rye bread	Mackerel pate (recipe 16) on rye bread with mixed salad	Salad with quinoa, mixed beans, cucumber, spring onion, sprouts	Cod with basil and lemon chickpeas	Wholegrain pitta bread with roast vegetables and hummus	Spicy carrot and lentil soup (recipe18); slice wholegrain bread	Wholegrain pitta pizza (recipe 19) with green salad
Mid-afternoon snack	Apple and 6 walnuts	Handful mixed nuts	Orange and small handful mixed nuts	Small tub probiotic yoghurt with berries	Handful mixed nuts	Vegetable sticks and hummus	Mug spicy carrot and lentil soup
Dinner	Warm prawn salad with lime soya dressing (recipe 20)	Vegetable chili (recipe 15) with quinoa	Cod with basil and lemon chickpeas (recipe 21)	Salmon fillets roast in oven with peppers, onions, courgettes & cherry tomatoes	Frittata made with roasted butternut squash, spinach and herbs with green salad (recipe 10)	Sea trout in a parcel with steamed vegetables (recipe 24)	Poached salmon with mustard herb sauce (recipe 22) and steamed vegetables

Some of you might prefer to see these meal suggestions as a list rather than in a table, so I have put week one in a list below:

Monday

Breakfast: Porridge made with water and berries, ground mixed seeds and a spoon of natural yoghurt

Mid-morning snack: Two oatcakes with thin spread hummus

Lunch: Carrot and chickpea soup

Mid-afternoon snack: Apple and seven almonds

Dinner: Asian salmon with steamed vegetables (recipe 23)

Tuesday

Breakfast: One slice wholemeal or rye toast and 1 poached or boiled egg

Mid-morning snack: Pear and small handful mixed nuts

Lunch: Tinned salmon mashed with probiotic yoghurt and salad

Mid-afternoon snack: Vegetable sticks with 1/3 tub hummus

Dinner: Quick tofu casserole with mixed vegetables (recipe 5)

Wednesday

Breakfast: Natural probiotic yoghurt with sugar-free muesli, berries, chopped nuts

Mid-morning snack: Two oatcakes with thin spread hummus

Lunch: Hard-boiled egg with avocado and mixed salad

Mid-afternoon snack: Small handful mixed nuts

Dinner: Healthy salmon burger with salad of lettuce, grated carrot, cucumber, scallion, tomato (recipe 6)

Thursday

Breakfast: Porridge with fruit compote and mixed chopped nuts (recipe 4)

Mid-morning snack: One wholegrain cracker with cottage cheese and cucumber

Lunch: Healthy salmon burger with mixed salad (recipe 6)

Mid-afternoon snack: Small tub natural probiotic yoghurt with handful berries

Dinner: Vegetable and prawn stir fry (recipe 13)

Friday

Breakfast: Muesli with oat milk, berries and mixed seeds (recipe 3)

Mid-morning snack: Small pot natural probiotic yoghurt with flaked almonds

Lunch: Vegetable and lentil soup (recipe 1)

Mid-afternoon snack: Orange and five brazil nuts

Dinner: Grilled mackerel with crunchy salad

Saturday

Breakfast: One slice wholemeal or rye toast with nut butter

Mid-morning snack: One wholegrain cracker with cottage cheese and cucumber

Lunch: Smoked or tinned mackerel and salad with watercress, spinach, cucumber and rocket

Mid-afternoon snack: Small handful mixed nuts

Dinner: Frittata made with roasted butternut squash, spinach and herbs with green salad

Sunday

Breakfast: Scrambled eggs and tomatoes or mushrooms on one slice rye toast

Mid-morning snack: Pear and handful mixed seeds

Lunch: Frittata made with roasted butternut squash, spinach and herbs with green salad (recipe 2)

Mid-afternoon snack: Vegetable sticks with 1/3 tub hummus

Dinner: Roast vegetable ratatouille with cod and butterbeans (recipe 7)

Out And About

You may need a quick lunch when you are out and about, and a sandwich often fits the bill. You might not have time to make your own at home but there are many places now where you can get some healthy choices.

Choose wholemeal bread, spelt, sourdough or rye. Wholemeal pitta can also make a change from sliced bread.

Suggestions for fillings if you are making your own and some of these you can get while out e.g. tuna and salad in wholemeal bread.

- Tahini and freshly sliced apple

- Hummus and salad

- Mashed avocado with a sprinkling of sunflower seeds

- Bean sprouts and tahini

- Tofu mashed with a little miso and salad

- Tuna and salad

- Miso, tahini, lettuce and a squeeze of lemon

- Egg and cress

- Avocado and salad

Eating Out

You may be eating out for some of your meals so think about the following:

- Remember the principle of combining protein with carbohydrates – you may be having white rice so have a smaller portion than you would have had before and load in up with extra vegetables or salad, along with the protein.

- Avoid foods which are almost pure carbohydrates (pizza, rissotto, pasta dishes, etc.)

- Where possible, choose a restaurant with some healthier options.

- Don't fill up on bread while waiting for the first course.

- Avoid meals with creamy or rich sauces and fried foods – especially deep fried foods in batter. Choose steamed or baked varieties instead.

- Ask for sauce on the side.

- Swap less healthy sides such as chips or white rice for steamed veg or tossed salad.

- Choose a starter and main or dessert and main, not both. Or have two starters instead of a starter and a main course.

- If you want a dessert, share it with someone else or have a fruit salad. But wait first, as it takes 20 minutes for your brain to register that you are full so you may not really need that dessert. Or would a cup of peppermint tea be OK instead?

Also, if you have been invited to a friend's house then you can still follow most of these principles above. If they are a close friend or family then you may be able to be a bit more prescriptive about what you are eating but, otherwise, I understand that you don't want to make someone feel awkward. So just reduce the portion of the carbohydrate on your plate or eat less of them, e.g. rice or potatoes, and eat more vegetables or salad. Cheese and biscuits would be a better choice instead of a dessert. There will probably be white flour crackers, but this is one of those 80/20 situations.

When Going Out For A Drink

- Be prepared!

- Try to eat at least a healthy snack before you go out and, if you know that it is going to be just drinks and very little food, then have something more substantail before you go that is slightly fatty, e.g. omelette to offset alcohol on an empty stomach.

- Or eat salted nuts or olives at a bar, but avoid other highly processed bar snacks.

• Alternate a glass of alcohol with a glass of water (sparkling with a twist of lemon or lime is a good going out alternative). Slowing down the amount of alcohol helps support your liver as well as your blood sugar.

When You Are On The Move

• Prepare yourself with portable, healthy snacks
  - Fruit and nuts.
  - Homemade energy bars/power balls, etc.
  - Flask of homemade soup or miso soup sachet.
  - Vegetable sticks and a pot of hummus.
  - Hard boiled egg, slice of frittata.
  - Bottle of water.

The Bottom Line

It is important to be prepared, especially when you are out. If your blood sugar drops because it is a long time since you last ate, your body will get a physiological urge for a quick fix and send you off for that coffee and Danish pastry. Remember, it is not because you are being weak-willed – it is your body trying to raise your blood sugar quickly (caffeine, sugar and white flour combination). But, if you have some nuts with you, aim to eat them before your blood sugar drops into hypoglycaemia so your body does not need that quick fix.

CHAPTER 23:

The role of stress

"Stress can make it difficult for a person with type 2 diabetes to control their blood sugar levels – and severe stress can cause insulin resistance even in people without diabetes."

I've talked a lot about how diet and nutrition can help to prevent or reverse type 2 diabetes, but there are other lifestyle factors to consider too – and I'm going to start with stress which, although not exactly a lifestyle choice, is something most of us live with – often without knowing it.

As I've already mentioned several times, stress can play a big part in the blood sugar roller coaster, so keeping it in check is vital to help prevent or reverse type 2 diabetes. And to do that, we need to understand exactly what stress is.

In fact, what we know as 'stress' is our body's natural 'fight or flight' response kicking in. We need this fight or flight response in dangerous or life-threatening situations, and it's what gives us that short, sharp burst of power to flee for our lives or find the strength to defend ourselves against an attacker. This was vital for our primitive ancestors who could have faced life or death situations on a daily basis – and it is exactly how the fight or flight response should be used by your body. The idea is that you would use your sudden energy burst to deal with the matter at hand. Then you'd calm down again.

It's an absolutely brilliant system that involves your brain registering a sense of danger and immediately stimulating the release of the stress hormones adrenaline and cortisol – and one role of these hormones is to release sugar into your blood so you have the energy to run or fight for your life.

The problem is that stress does not just come from life threatening situations. These days it is more likely to come from emotionally challenging events. And, clever though your brain is, it has not evolved to distinguish between stress that arises from mortal danger and the kind of stress that comes from being up against a deadline, or stuck in a traffic jam.

So, the same hormones are released in response to stresses and strains of everyday life. And, because these kinds of stresses tend to be chronic – often going on for weeks or months – there is no let-up in the release of these hormones. You are not running away or fighting, so you don't need the burst of blood sugar and energy that cortisol has given you. Instead, the sugar remains in your blood – and, for as long as your stress persists, you will carry on releasing excess cortisol and suffering the consequences of high blood sugar levels. Your insulin levels are dampened in order to keep your blood sugar high (because your body mistakenly thinks it needs this) and this, essentially, makes your cells insulin resistant. With chronic stress, cortisol is sending the same message out all the time. Your pancreas desperately tries to produce more insulin – and your blood glucose will stay high because the glucose can't get into your cells... and so it goes on, in a vicious cycle.

If your body is producing too much cortisol, you may feel some of the following symptoms:

- **Weakness And Fatigue**

Cortisol imbalances can throw off your body's blood sugar metabolism, making you feel weak, tired and run-down. Too much cortisol can also interfere with sleep patterns and produce a 'wakeful' unrelaxing sleep state. When this happens, you may feel worn-out even after a full night's sleep.

- **Muscle And Joint Pain**

Excess cortisol in the bloodstream accelerates the breakdown of body tissue and prevents proper tissue repair, leading to muscle and joint injuries and chronic pain.

- **Obesity**

Cortisol imbalances can stimulate fat deposits in various parts of the body, resulting in weight gains in the trunk, chest, neck, and face.

- **Poor Skin**

High levels of cortisol can reduce your skin's ability to regenerate, resulting in an unhealthy skin appearance.

Over time, cortisol imbalances can take a heavy toll on your health, wearing down your immune system, triggering premature ageing, and setting the stage for chronic illness. Anxiety, depression, heart disease and osteoporosis have all been linked with elevated cortisol levels.

It is well known that stress can make it difficult for a person with type 2 diabetes to control their blood sugar levels – and severe stress can cause insulin resistance even in people without diabetes, and also change how your pancreas functions.[240]

Financial downturn, bereavement, work pressures and family trauma can all set off the stress response – and, once triggered, your own behaviour may inadvertently perpetuate your stress, so your stress hormones remain high, even when the initial shock has passed. In fact, the feeling of being stressed may become so familiar and normal to you that you are not actually aware that stress is an issue. Because this is such a common scenario, it's worth reminding yourself of the symptoms of chronic stress. You may be surprised at how wide ranging and seemingly random they are.

These symptoms include:

- Sleep problems (which I will discuss in detail in the next chapter)

- Back, neck and head pain from tense muscles

- Digestive disorders

- Hair loss

- Fatigue

- High blood pressure
- Palpitations
- Chest pain
- Skin problems (hives, eczema and other rashes)
- Jaw pain (from grinding your teeth)
- Sexual difficulties
- Recurrent colds and infections
- Nervousness, anxiety and panic attacks
- Depression and moodiness
- Irritability and frustration
- Memory problems and lack of concentration

To make the vicious cycle even worse, stress changes how you eat and the food choices you make, so you're more likely to reach for those comforting sugary foods. This is because, after stress hormones have been released, your body thinks you have either run or fought for your life. Now it believes it needs to refuel and restock – just in case there is going to be another life-threatening event coming around the corner. Hence it will increase your appetite to hoard calories because the next stress may be a famine – so it will send you off for those quick fixes to restock your energy stores quickly.[241]

DHEA

DHEA (dehydroepiandrosterone) is another hormone produced by your adrenal glands that works to balance many of the negative effects of cortisol and helps you cope better with stress. When cortisol and DHEA are chronically *'out of sync'*, they can tax your body's immune system, making you less able to cope with stress and more susceptible to a wide range of illnesses. That is why it is so important to get cortisol under control.

In some countries, like America, DHEA is sold as a food supplement but in the UK it is only available on prescription and rightly so. DHEA is a steroid hormone and the body easily converts it into oestrogen and testosterone, so it must be used with extreme caution in anyone with a hormonal cancer. Other noted side effects are palpitations, excess growth of body hair and also hair loss (male pattern baldness). In the UK, DHEA is classed as an unlicensed medicine, meaning that it does not have a product licence from the Medicine and Healthcare products Regulatory Agency (MHRA) and is, therefore, not proven to be safe and effective. In the UK, DHEA can only be given as a private prescription.

Although we know that our food selection definitely changes under stress, interestingly it seems that women are more likely than men not just to eat more food in general when they're stressed, but to also reach for the very foods that they would normally avoid because they know they are unhealthy. Research shows that we are eating these foods in order to feel better – however I think there is also an evolutionary benefit reaching back to when we led lives that were fraught with jeopardy most of the time, with the frequent threat of famine as well as the danger of wild animals.[242]

You might have the feeling that a sweet 'comfort food' will calm you down. But we also have a tendency to reach for the same comfort foods when we're bored, lonely, angry or sad. Ask yourself which emotion you are trying to dampen down with sugar. Can you try to find an activity that actually deals with the emotion, rather than squashing it down? Talking to a friend could help, or consider seeing a counsellor or therapist to get to the bottom of your feelings of anger or sadness.

At work, try to devise strategies to reduce the amount of stress you are under – asking for help, delegating, and learning to say no are all good ways to start. If your job is stressing you a lot, can you change it – if not completely, then in small but significant ways (reduce your hours, move department, work from home for part of the week)?

Likewise, if friends are overloading you, can you take a step back? Without positive action, no treatment plan will be as effective as it could be.

Added to the blood sugar issues, stress also changes your body shape, as I mentioned on page 32, and it causes weight to pile on around your middle.

This is really important as it is clear that even if you are a normal weight (normal BMI) but have fat around your middle then this alone can increase your risk of type 2 diabetes by causing insulin resistance. The fat stores around your middle are an easy source of energy when the fight or flight response is triggered – but of course, these days, you may not need to use the fat stores for the same purposes as your ancestors did.

Are You Stressed? Take The Test…

Do you find it difficult to get up in the mornings? Have your periods stopped or become irregular? Are you constantly under pressure and/or overloaded? A wide range of physical and emotional disorders have been linked to stress which, in turn, can relate to adrenal hormone imbalances.

Ask yourself the following questions:

- Do you often feel weak and tired, for no apparent reason?

- Are you under chronic stress?

- Do you have trouble getting a night of restful sleep?

- Do you have low sex drive?

- Are you exposed to high noise levels?

- Are you feeling anxious or depressed?

- Do you have menstrual difficulties?

- Are you suffering from joint pain?

- Do you have an eating disorder?

- Have you recently gained or lost weight?

- Do you suffer from ulcers or irritable bowel syndrome?

- Do you have trouble with concentration, memory or learning?

- Do you suffer from hypertension?

If you answered yes to any of these questions, you may be suffering from an over- or under-reactive stress response by your adrenal hormones.

There is also an Adrenal Stress Test, that measures both cortisol and DHEA, that you can take to find out how stressed you are – see full details in Chapter 26.

Controlling Stress

You can never totally avoid stress, because it is triggered by such a huge range of psychological factors and external events. You can become stressed by relationships, work, finances, and even by social interactions and how you perceive yourself on social media. Obviously, some of these can be controlled by looking within yourself – but not everything in modern life can be controlled, and you may conclude that you can't control the stress in your life.

Even if this is the case, you can control how it affects you physically, and you can make sure you are not exacerbating it. For example, there is a chance that your pattern of eating is subconsciously telling your body that it is under even more stress – but, by taking control of your blood sugar roller coaster with the dietary recommendations in chapter 7, you will stop your body from releasing such high levels of stress hormones and will automatically feel calmer in yourself.

Make sure you have eliminated caffeine (including coffee, tea, chocolate, colas, energy drinks) and all other stimulants (including alcohol and cigarettes), as one effect of stimulants is to make you feel more stressed. And, while thinking about the importance of what you eat, and also when you eat, as discussed in earlier chapters, do remember that this is not the time to fast. Because, as far as your body is concerned, fasting is a stress. When you miss meals, you are signalling to your brain that there is a shortage of food and a threat to your survival. It is a matter of life or death. So, if you are already stressed or fatigued, adding a further stress to your body by fasting could be severely damaging to health.

Meditation, mindfulness, tai chi, qi gong and yoga can all help control stress.

There are many different ways to meditate – from repeating a mantra in your head, to focusing on your breath or following a guided meditation that takes your imagination on a journey. Studies show that meditation has both short-term and long-term benefits, and mindfulness works in a similar way, by focusing your mind on a specific activity and really experiencing the moment that you're in. It's a way of distracting yourself from everyday stresses, and can be practiced during the most mundane of daily chores such as washing up or sorting laundry.

Yoga, tai chi and qi gong all involve slow, controlled movements with a focus on breathing correctly, which can be very calming. As such, they reduce stress and lower levels of cortisol, which helps with your fat-loss programme. Yoga, in particular, is useful for changing the way that you breathe. At times of stress, many of us will shallow breathe without realising it, and this can exacerbate our stress and lead to hyperventilation and even panic attacks. Slow, deep breathing is a key element of yoga practice, and a handy tool to return to whenever you feel stress mounting. It calms the sympathetic nervous system (the part linked to your fight or flight response). (Conversely, shallow breathing – hyperventilating – can make you feel more anxious.)

Learn To Breathe

Unlike a baby, whose whole abdomen rises and falls as they breathe (because they are breathing with their diaphragm) most adults tend to shallow-breathe using just the top half of their chest – and this makes them more tense and also tired.

By learning to breathe with your diaphragm (belly-breathing), you will not only be signalling to your body that you are less stressed, but you will also be circulating more oxygen around your body and mind. This will give you more energy, allow the feel-good neurotransmitters in the brain to do their job efficiently and also activate the relaxation centres in the brain.

Do You Shallow-Breathe Or Belly-Breathe?

Lie down on your back. Put your right hand on your chest and your left hand over your belly button. Breathe as you would normally. Watch your hands and see which one moves more with each breath. If the right hand is moving more than the left you are a shallow- (or chest-) breather and this needs to change.

Start with this simple exercise for 10 minutes each day over the next week:

1. Lie on your stomach with your legs approximately 60cm (2ft) apart and your feet relaxed outwards.

2. Fold your arms, place your hands on your biceps and your head on your arms.

3. Relax.

Because of the pressure from the floor, you will only be able to breathe through your diaphragm, so just feel your breathing for the next 10 minutes:

- Your breath should flow smoothly in and out.

- The out-breath should be longer than the in-breath.

- You should be breathing through your nose and not your mouth.

Once you have the done this 10 minutes daily for a week, try it standing upright:

1. Stand with your feet slightly apart.

2. Take a few gentle breaths in and out through your nose.

3. Place your hands over your belly.

4. As you breathe in, push your belly out – you should be able to feel your hands being pushed out.

5. Pause briefly.

6. Breathe out slowly through your nose.

7. As you breathe out, imagine all the tension and stress leaving your body just like a soft flowing stream.

8. Repeat 10 times.

Try to do this every day over the next three months.

Important Nutrients For Stress

Some nutrients have a special role to play in helping to reduce stress levels. When you are under stress you use up a lot of your B vitamins – especially vitamins B2 and B5 – as well as vitamin C.

Stress depletes your stores of vitamin C. Animals that can manufacture their own vitamin C, in the liver and kidneys, do so when they are stressed, replenishing stocks to restore health. But, because the human body can't make its own vitamin C, you need to make sure that, during times of anxiety, you supplement your own stocks – not only by eating more vitamin C rich foods, but also adding in a supplement.

Vitamin C and the B vitamins are all water-soluble vitamins, so you need to eat them in your diet on a day-to-day basis (or get them from food supplements), because your body doesn't store them. The best sources of all the B vitamins are whole grains, green leafy vegetables, and nuts and seeds.

The other nutrient that prolonged stress depletes is magnesium, a calming mineral often referred to as 'nature's tranquilliser'. It helps to relieve anxiety and relax muscles. One common symptom of magnesium deficiency is waking up in the early hours of the morning and not being able to get back to sleep. Increase your intake of green leafy vegetables, nuts and seeds to boost your magnesium levels.

As well as magnesium and B vitamins, there are other supplements that are good for restoring your sense of calm.

- Siberian ginseng. This regulates the production of cortisol and acts as a tonic to your adrenal glands. It is an adaptogen, which means it can help your body to adapt in any way it needs in order to cope with stress. It also helps with energy levels, stamina and endurance – and it can boost immunity, too.

- L-theanine. This amino acid is found in some green teas. It helps transmit nerve impulses in the brain and reduces stress and anxiety.

There is a supplement I use in the clinic by NHP called Tranquil Support which can be very helpful if stress is an issue for you (see www.naturalhealthpractice.com).

The Bottom Line

Stress affects most of us at some point in our lives. The key is to get to know the tell-tale signs and take control before it takes control of you – because living with too much stress will undoubtedly impact on your health and increase your risk of type 2 diabetes.

CHAPTER 24:

The importance of sleep

"Three nights of poor sleep can have the same effect on your body's ability to control blood sugar levels as putting on more than two stone in weight."

Very closely linked to stress, is sleep – or rather the lack of it. And that matters, because we now know that not getting enough sleep increases your risk of both being overweight and developing type 2 diabetes. You're also at greater risk of cancer and Alzheimer's if you don't sleep well.

This is all relatively new knowledge, though. The research is only just beginning to catch up with us and, for those who pride themselves on getting by with minimal hours in bed, it may be difficult to accept that how we sleep is actually just as vital as our diet and exercise regimes to our health and wellbeing.

When you don't get enough good quality sleep, you can feel irritable, foggy brained and, of course, tired. But, beneath the surface, so much more will be going on – because it is while you are asleep that your body can recharge its batteries and repair its cells and tissues.

And yet, despite its critical role, sleep is too often perceived as something of a luxury – because the less we sleep, the more we can pack into our ever more busy days. In fact, since the 1900s the average time we sleep each night has dropped from nine to seven and a half hours – but, by depriving ourselves of sleep, we may find that we are not as productive the next day. And, as I've mentioned above, that lack of sleep will also have long-term consequences for our health.

As you know, when you're stressed you produce the hormones adrenaline and cortisol. But cortisol also has a circadian rhythm, meaning that its levels naturally fluctuate over the course of 24 hours.

Levels should be highest when you wake in the morning, revving you up ready to start the day. Then, towards the end of the day, levels should naturally decline, so they're at their lowest during the night.

The action of cortisol is almost the direct opposite of another hormone, melatonin. Known as your sleep hormone, levels of melatonin are highest at night and then fall off to their lowest levels by the morning. However, if you are stressed and your cortisol levels stay high, melatonin production stays low, making it hard for you to go to sleep. This is an extremely common scenario: one in three people are affected by insomnia which can mean difficulty in getting to sleep and/or waking during the night and not being able to get back to sleep.

The Stages Of Sleep

There are two different types of sleep – REM (rapid eye movement) and non-REM sleep and there are different stages within these types.

During the night we cycle through four different stages before we wake up. But we don't progress through these stages in sequence. Instead, your sleep begins in stage one and then goes into stages two and three. After that, stage two is repeated and then you go into stage four REM sleep. Then you go back to stage two. You can go through this cycle about five times during the night. Each time you go into REM sleep it gets longer.

Stage 1 – is that changeover between wakefulness and sleep. It is light non-REM sleep and lasts about five to 10 minutes.

Stage 2 – is also non-REM sleep and your body temperature will drop, and your heart rate will slow.

Stage 3 – is also non-REM sleep and when the deepest sleep occurs. Your breathing slows to its lowest rate and it is this kind of sleep that makes you feel refreshed in the morning.

Stage 4 – this is REM sleep and the first time you experience it is about 90 minutes after you fall asleep. Your eyes can move rapidly from side to side underneath your closed eyelids. This is the stage when most of your dreaming can occur.

Why Is Sleep So Important For Type 2 Diabetes?

Research has shown that if you are sleep deprived you could end up putting on weight and, as I've shown, being overweight increases your risk of type 2 diabetes. This is partly because being sleep deprived reduces your levels of the appetite-controlling hormone leptin while increasing your levels of ghrelin (the hormone that makes you want to eat more and is thought to play a role in the long-term regulation of your body weight). One large study of nearly 70,000 women, over 16 years, found that those who slept less than five hours a night gained more weight over time than those who slept for seven hours a night.[243]

But disrupted sleep also affects your body's metabolism and reduces its ability to convert sugar into energy – and this heightens your risk of diabetes. In fact, just three nights of poor sleep can have the same effect on your body's ability to control blood sugar levels as putting on more than two stone in weight.[244]

Sleeping for less than five hours a night greatly increases your risk of type 2 diabetes.[245] But, by changing your sleep pattern, you can actually improve your blood sugar control and reduce the effects of type 2 diabetes.[246]

It is the deepest slow wave sleep – the third stage – that seems to be the most restorative sleep and it's during this state that hormonal changes occur and alter glucose regulation. Research has shown that if stage 3 is suppressed in healthy young adults, without shortening their overall sleep time, there is a marked decrease in insulin sensitivity.[247] The thinking is that the reduction in this stage of sleep could also be what increases the risk of type 2 diabetes, when stage 3 sleep naturally declines as we get older. Stage 3 sleep is also reduced by obesity and being overweight, partly because being overweight increases your risk of the sleep disorder Obstructive Sleep Apnoea – and this seems to affect slow wave sleep.

There are many other repercussions of poor sleep too:

- **Good sleep helps you look and feel better:** People who have less than five hours sleep a night tend to have more physical ailments, such as headaches and stomach upsets; and they also undergo changes in metabolism similar to those that normally seem to occur as part of the ageing process. When you're fast asleep, your body goes into repair mode and regenerates your skin, blood and brain cells, as well as your muscles. Small wonder that many of us look worse for wear after a poor night's sleep! You can spend a fortune on anti-ageing skin creams, but you need to sleep well to have healthy, glowing skin.

- **Good sleep helps to protect your cardiovascular system:** Research shows that those who sleep five hours or less a night are twice as likely to suffer from hypertension (high blood pressure),[248] and a large study of nearly 500,000 adults with no previous cardiovascular risk showed that those who slept less than six hours a night has a 20% increase risk of heart attack over a seven year period.[249]

- **Good sleep helps your immune system:** Research has shown that missing even a few hours a night on a regular basis can decrease the number of 'natural killer cells', which are responsible for fighting off invaders such as bacteria and viruses.[250] As your immune system can also alter your sleep, which can, in turn, affect your immune function, this is another vicious cycle.[251]

When you get the seasonal flu, all you want to do is sleep – because your body innately knows that it is during sleep that your immune defences are able to be more effectively mobilised.

Seven hours of sleep a night enhances the function of T cells, a type of white blood cell which attacks and kills viruses, and one study showed that, when people were actively given the common cold virus, those who'd had less sleep were more likely to be infected and 'catch a cold'. For those sleeping five hours a night the infection rate was nearly 50%. For those sleeping seven hours a night it was just 18%.[252]

And, when two groups of people were given the flu vaccine, one group having four hours sleep, the other seven hours, the group with only four hours of sleep produced only half the level of protected antibodies to the flu virus. So, the amount of sleep actually changed how their bodies responded to the vaccine.[253]

None of this will come as any surprise to those of you who succumb to colds and other illnesses when you are run down – normally after periods of inadequate sleep.

• **Good sleep makes you smarter:** Those with sleep deprivation suffer from reduced concentration and memory loss, and they are more likely to make mistakes and have a slower reaction time. And night owls beware! A study found that people who slept after learning and practising a new task remembered more about it the following day than people who stayed up all night learning the same thing.[254] Better sleep means better concentration and better decision-making.

• **Good sleep makes you a nicer person:** The most potent effects of sleep deprivation are on our behaviour. Lack of sleep will make you cranky, aggressive, forgetful and unsociable. Taken to extremes, severe sleep deprivation causes depression, disorientation and paranoia.

• **Good sleep helps prevent Alzheimer's:** Sleep is necessary to help consolidate the effects of your waking experience; it converts your memories into more permanent and enhanced forms so that it is easier to retrieve them. This aspect of sleep is really important as Alzheimer's is now called type 3 diabetes. Too little sleep increases your risk for Alzheimer's because beta-amyloid protein is cleared away during sleep when your cerebrospinal fluid washes out toxins from your body.

Interestingly, research on mice has shown that the cerebrospinal detoxification process only happens when a mouse is sleeping. As soon as the mouse goes to sleep, the cerebrospinal fluid floods through its brain. At the same time, brain cells seem to shrink, making space for the fluid to flow freely through and around them, taking out the waste. This process does not happen when the mouse is awake.

So, what happens if you're not sleeping well? We know that in mice who have been bred to model Alzheimer's, sleep deprivation causes a substantial increase in beta-amyloid plaque build-up. And when researchers have looked at older people without Alzheimer's, those who are sleeping for shorter amounts of time and have poor-quality sleep have more beta-amyloid plaque build-up.[255]

Getting adequate amounts of good-quality sleep is crucial (aim for six to eight hours uninterrupted sleep every night). And the position in which you sleep can also be a factor. When you sleep on your side, your body seems more able to remove the build-up of so-called 'brain waste' chemicals, such as beta-amyloid proteins, that are thought to contribute to this and other neurological diseases such as Parkinson's.[256]

Routine Matters

If you are not already sleeping well, you should look at your bedtime routine. Poor 'sleep hygiene' is the most common cause of insomnia and disturbed sleep. Your busy, active brain needs to be treated like a dimmer switch and allowed to wind down slowly. Ideally, you should allow about 40 minutes to switch off with whatever relaxing routine you find most helpful – for example, having a bath, reading, or listening to an audio book. But, before you do any of that, you need to switch off your TV, phone and tablet – at least an hour (ideally two) before you intend to go to bed.

This is not just about bombarding your brain with information just before you try to sleep, there are physical factors at work: backlit screens, such as those of a tablet or smartphone, emit blue light that interferes with your body's production of melatonin – the hormone that regulates your body's circadian rhythm, the 24-hour rhythm of day and night.[257]

As it goes, exposure to bright light of any colour before bed will suppress your melatonin production – it's just that blue light is worst of all. Studies show that sitting in bright light, compared to a dim light, delays melatonin onset and shortens melatonin exposure by up to 90 minutes – that is, it takes a full hour and a half for the effects of bright-light exposure to wear off and melatonin to kick in and make you feel sleepy. If you leave your bedroom light on when you're sleeping, your melatonin secretion will be suppressed by more than 50%.[258] Unsurprisingly, then, researchers suggest that *'chronically exposing oneself to electrical lighting in the late evening disrupts melatonin signalling and could therefore potentially impact not only sleep, but also thermoregulation (our ability to control our temperature), blood pressure, and glucose homeostasis'.*

The amount of light you are exposed to before bed can also change how much fat you burn while you are asleep. A recent study exposed people to bright or dim light before falling asleep. The researchers found that those exposed to bright light experienced a significant reduction in their ability to burn fat while they slept. This means that using devices before bedtime can make it much harder to lose weight or may even cause weight gain.[259] In another large study in 2019, following over 43,000 women for six years, those who slept with a light on had higher levels of obesity.[260] This information is so important in controlling type 2 diabetes.

It is also not a good idea to have a large meal at the end of the day, close to bedtime, because your digestive system should be winding down and it is going to struggle to digest your food efficiently. You can then end up with indigestion or heartburn which will affect our sleep. And try and keep to having two to three hours with no food between your last meal and going to bed, so no after dinner snacking except for a couple of weeks if you are trying to stop waking up at 3 or 4am (see page 208).

Herbs That Help With Sleep

There are some very good traditional herbs that have been used for centuries to help with sleep problems. These include valerian, chamomile, hops, lemon balm and passionflower. Valerian has been shown to reduce the time it takes to fall asleep by 15 to 20 minutes and to improve sleep quality.[261] And it is even more effective when it's combined with other herbs such as hops and lemon balm.

Chamomile has calming effects and contains an antioxidant called apigenin which binds to specific receptors in the brain to decrease anxiety and help to initiate sleep.[262]

Lemon balm has been used with stressed volunteers who were experiencing anxiety disorders and sleep disturbances. It not only helped them sleep better but also reduced their anxiety.[263] Seventy per cent of the volunteers achieved full remission from anxiety, 85% for insomnia and 70% for both.

Passionflower is helpful for sleep problems and, when combined with valerian and hops, was as effective as an insomnia medication (zolpidem) at improving sleep quality.[264]

Hops are also helpful, especially when combined with valerian, in reducing the amount of time it takes to get off to sleep, increasing the amount of time spent asleep and also lessening night awakening.[265]

The amino acid l-theanine is really helpful if you feel 'tired but wired'; where you are exhausted but as soon as your head hits the pillow your brain is very active and doesn't allow you to fall asleep.

There has also been good research on tart cherries which has shown that these have helped people with insomnia increase sleep time by up to 84 minutes.[266] Interestingly, tart cherries have been shown to increase melatonin and to have a beneficial effect on both sleep duration and quality.[267] Other benefits of tart cherries include reducing inflammation, blood pressure, arthritis and exercise-induced muscle soreness, as well as reducing HbA1c.[268]

I use NHP's Advanced Sleep Support in my clinics which contains all the nutrients and herbs mentioned above (see www. naturalhealthpractice.com).

Use Relaxation Or Visualisation Techniques

If you find that your mind will not shut off then you need to retrain it to calm down as you go to bed. Sometimes the easiest way to do this, especially if you have an active mind or are a 'worrier', is to get your mind to think of something else. Take yourself off to a wonderful beach or a beautiful garden and let all your senses become involved. Hear the sounds on that beach, smell the flowers in the garden, feel the sand through your toes, picture the blue sky, and really make the place come alive. Each night that you do this, you will find that the time it takes to go to sleep will get shorter and shorter because going to this beautiful place signals to your brain that this is the time for sleep.

Do You Wake At 3 Or 4am?

This can be a common problem for many people. You might be one of the lucky ones that go back to sleep easily if you wake but it's not unusual to be awake for an hour to two after having woken up, and this then has a knock-on effect on your energy and wellbeing the next day.

You can be producing adrenaline and cortisol on that rollercoaster of blood sugar that is described on page 66 and that goes on day and night. This means that you can get an adrenaline surge in the middle of the night – because your blood sugar has dropped – and this will wake you up. You could just be wide awake, or you could wake up sweating, or with your mind racing. And you could even have palpitations.

It is important that you follow the recommendations on page 162 to keep your blood sugar in balance during the day and, for only a couple of weeks while you are changing your diet, have a small snack of complex carbohydrates – maybe an oat cake, or half a slice of wheat or rye bread – about an hour before bed. This will stop your blood sugar dropping overnight and prevent adrenaline from being released into your bloodstream and causing you to wake.

Make The Most Of Tryptophan

Your body needs the amino acid tryptophan in order to make serotonin, the relaxing and calming brain neurotransmitter. Many antidepressants, like Prozac, are called Selective Serotonin Reuptake Inhibitors (SSRI) and they work by helping to keep serotonin levels high in the brain.

Tryptophan occurs naturally in certain foods, which are good to include in your evening meal to help you sleep. It is one of a number of amino acids broken down from the protein that you eat, but it is outnumbered by the other amino acids and tryptophan molecules may not get into your brain, because they are competing with the other amino acids to get through. The key is to always combine protein with carbohydrate to keep your blood sugar levels stable, as this changes everything. The insulin released when you eat carbohydrates is used by the other amino acids and that means that the tryptophan can get across the blood/brain barrier.

Tryptophan containing foods include:

Fish

Whole grains

Beans like soya, chickpeas

Almonds

Peanuts

Eggs

Bananas

Dates

Dairy

Combine these with a carbohydrate, but remember to avoid carbohydrates that are refined and have a high glycaemic index. These can cause too much insulin to be produced during the night, leading your blood sugar to drop (hypoglycaemia) and waking you up in the early hours. Just a small amount of good quality, unrefined carbohydrate should be eaten in the evening.

The Effects Of Sleeping Pills

If you are not sleeping well, is it a good idea to take sleeping pills? The straightforward answer is no – you should attempt to really avoid them if you can and try the natural remedies on page 207 beforehand. That said, it is thought that one in 10 people are regularly taking a drug to help them sleep.

In 2006, Forbes magazine published an article called The Sleep Racket which showed the billions that people are spending on pillows, mattresses, humidifiers, bath soaks, etc. every year. And now we have apps and other digital tools designed to help you sleep better.

Sleeping pills do seem like the quick-fix solution to what has now been termed an epidemic, but you can become dependent on them and they can even become addictive. And you are not really addressing the underlying cause of why you are not sleeping, so if you come off them the problem is still there.

One class of sleeping medication, benzodiazepines (which includes flurazepam, loprazolam, lormetazepam and nitrazepam), reduces the amount of Stage 3 deep slow wave sleep that you get – and remember this is the most restorative part of sleep and that this is the stage of sleep that seems to have the biggest impact on your risk of type 2 diabetes.

Other sleeping medications known as Z drugs – zaleplon, eszopiclone and zolpidem – do not have the same effect on your stages of sleep. But they only seem to increase your length of sleep by 12 minutes.[269]

Perhaps the most alarming aspect of sleeping medication, as research in *The BMJ* has suggested, is that they can increase your risk of death fourfold, by increasing your risk of cancer and heart disease.[270]

Top Tips For A Good Night's Sleep

As well as putting away screens one to two hours before you go to bed and creating a relaxing bedtime routine, try adopting the following as part of your good sleep hygiene:

- Use blackout curtains or blinds, which can stop morning light waking you too early and will help to mask the light of bright streetlights, if you have them, outside your bedroom window. Or use an eye mask if easier.

- Don't have an alarm clock or any device that emits a light during the night.

- If you need a night light (for example, to light your way to the toilet), then use a dim, red light, as this bypasses your optic nerves in such a way as not to interfere with your body's production of melatonin.

- Get lots of bright light during the day and early evening, as this will help improve your sleep and melatonin levels.[271]

- Keep your bedroom cooler rather than warmer, then layer on blankets that you can add or remove during the night if you get too cold or hot.

- Use cotton bedding, which will enable your body to regulate your temperature more effectively during the night, improving your ability to sleep through.

- Invest in a comfortable mattress – the best and most comfortable you can afford!

- Try and go to bed at the same time each day.

And also try these other natural solutions for better sleep:

- Take vitamin C to keep your stress hormones in check.

- Take probiotics to help your body produce serotonin (vital for making the hormone melatonin).

- Add in magnesium and lemon balm to help relax your body.

- Try using the herbs valerian and passionflower, which can influence certain brain chemicals to calm your mind and help you relax.

- Try homeopathy, opting for *Chamomilla* if you're feeling tired but can't get off to sleep; *Cocculus* for insomnia caused by mental and physical exhaustion; *Coffea* if you've too many thoughts running through your head; or *Arnica* if you're overtired and restless.

- Use aromatherapy. Spritz your pillow with lavender or melissa, or massage one or other of these oils (check for suitable dilutions, as necessary) into your temples and pulse points. Or you could have a warm bath before bed using aromatherapy oils such as bergamot, lavender, roman chamomile or marjoram.

- Avoid anything that has a stimulant effect such as caffeine, chocolate (especially dark chocolate). And of course the closer to bedtime, the worse the effect. For some people it is better not to have any caffeine after midday as some people are very sensitive to it causing sleep problems.

- Alcohol can also change your sleep pattern as you don't get such deep sleep and can wake easily. It also acts as a diuretic so you will need to get up to pass urine. Alcohol also stops the passage of tryptophan into your brain (see page 209) and it is this amino acid which is converted into serotonin, your 'feel good' brain chemical.

- Exercise during the day can help you sleep better but avoid exercise near bedtime as it can be stimulating. Exercise can also delay the production of melatonin, which is known to help with sleep.

Melatonin Supplementation

As we've already seen, the function of melatonin is crucial for a good night's sleep,

So wouldn't it be wonderful if we could take it as a supplement? In fact, it used to be available in tablets in health food shops in the UK (and in the USA it still is), but I would not recommend using it without medical supervision: it is a hormone, not a nutrient, so I believe it should be prescribed by a medical practitioner. In the UK, it is classed as an unlicensed medicine and does not have a product licence so would need to be given on a private prescription.

Taking one hormone is likely to affect the balance of other hormones in your system, because your hormones work in a feedback loop – one triggering changes in the levels of another to make up your whole endocrine system.

I believe it's much better to address the underlying causes of your sleep problems (whether they are a result of stress, poor sleep hygiene or another cause), so that you restore balance throughout your body, as well as restoring good sleep.

Furthermore, melatonin supplementation comes with side-effects, including daytime sleepiness, headaches, dizziness, irritability, depression and stomach cramps.

There is also conflicting evidence as to whether melatonin is helpful or harmful in relation to type 2 diabetes risk and whether it increases or decreases fasting glucose and glucose tolerance.[272]

A Word About Shift Work

All of this information on sleep is helpful but, of course, it is very different if you are having to go against your natural circadian rhythm of night and day because you are working shifts.

Unfortunately, shift work in itself puts you more at risk of a higher range of health problems, including weight gain, heart disease, peptic ulcers and an inability to control your blood sugar levels,[273] which results in an increased risk of weight gain and type 2 diabetes. A large-scale meta-analysis of over 226,00 people suggests that the increased risk of type 2 diabetes is as high as 42%, especially for those on rotating day and night shifts.[274]

It is thought that some of these problems may be linked to the quality of food choices, as it may be easier to go for instant meals, and also the irregular times of eating. And we know that the disruption in sleep can affect blood sugar levels. It had been thought that being on a schedule of permanent night shifts[275] (rather than rotating shifts) could minimise the health problems as your circadian rhythm would adjust over time – but, unfortunately, this doesn't seem to be the case.

CHAPTER 25:

Keeping active

"Exercise really comes into its own for pre-diabetes, type 2 diabetes and their prevention."

Everybody talks about exercise and how important it is for your general health and that is definitely true. It's the equivalent of a wonder drug, boosting the health of your heart, bowels and immune system. It lifts your mood, reduces stress and anxiety, builds strong bones, lowers blood pressure and even cuts your risk of breast and colon cancers.

But it really comes into its own for prediabetes, type 2 diabetes and their prevention.[276] It lowers your blood sugar levels and HbA1c, and it improves your insulin sensitivity and has been shown to lower type 2 diabetes risk by up to 58% in high-risk people.

Long term research over 13 years from the Diabetes Prevention Programme has shown that diabetes incidence was significantly lower in those who exercised, compared to a placebo group, and the difference could not be explained by changes in weight alone.[277]

Exercise improves insulin sensitivity by up to 50% and this benefit can last for as long as 72 hours after the last exercise session[278] and that is why regular exercise is so important. As I mentioned on page 23, as well as being insulin resistant you can become leptin resistant – meaning that your calls cannot use the hormone leptin, which controls your appetite and hunger. But the more you exercise, the more your cells stay sensitive to leptin and the less you are at risk of diabetes.[279]

It is thought that insulin resistant muscles may be the starting point of type 2 diabetes – and muscles can become insulin resistant years before your start having problems with your blood sugar.[280]

Your muscles take 80% of the glucose (energy) you get after eating – and they take in the glucose without using insulin, so it doesn't matter if you are not producing enough insulin or even if you are insulin resistant. Your muscles can still reduce the amount of glucose in your blood. They need glucose for energy when you exercise and this helps your insulin receptors stay sensitive to insulin.

And, although many of us have been raised to believe we shouldn't exercise straight after eating, the science now suggests that going for a moderate walk after a meal can be particularly helpful for balancing your blood sugar. One study showed that people who ate two slices of white bread and then went for a walk lowered their blood sugar levels more than those who walked before eating the bread. Walking at a slow pace for 15 minutes after eating results in a 1.5mmol/L reduction in blood glucose.[281] And, for those with type 2 diabetes, walking for 10 minutes after each meal lowered blood sugar levels more effectively than walking for 30 minutes at any other time of the day.[282]

Maybe you haven't exercised for a while and are reluctant to go to the gym or join in classes – just walking can be very beneficial for your health and diabetes. I would suggest you start slowly – especially if you are overweight – and then increase both the duration of the walk and the intensity – enough to get slightly out of breath. If time is short, you can break up the time into smaller amounts instead of aiming for, say, 30 minutes in one go.

A huge study of over 33,000 runners and 15,000 walkers has shown that walking briskly can lower your risk of diabetes and also high blood pressure and cholesterol just as much as running, when the same amount of energy is used. The researchers compared the runners and walkers over the same distance with, of course, different intensities. But it showed that the walkers got just as many benefits over 5k as the runners. It just took them longer to cover the distance.[283] Walking is much easier on your joints than running and it also helps to reduce stress because running can increase cortisol.

Walking, and especially brisk walking, helps to build muscles and can also help to target the fat around your middle (visceral fat), which produces toxic substances that increase your risk of type 2 diabetes. When you are fast walking (which is classed as a low to moderate intensity exercise), you are burning fat. Conversely, a vigorous activity like running will use carbohydrates.

This shows that walking is a good activity for you and the further you can walk each time the better.

The American Diabetes Association suggests that, in order to maintain insulin sensitivity,[284] people with type 2 diabetes should take at least 150 minutes a week of moderate to vigorous activity and not to allow more than two days to elapse between activity sessions.

And not only can walking help with type 2 diabetes, but you are also reducing your risk of severe COVID-19 and death. But the speed with which you walk also makes a difference. If you are a slow walker (under 3mph) you are 2.5 times more likely to develop severe COVID and 3.75 times more likely to die from it than faster walkers – even if, as a slow walker, you are a healthy weight.[285] You are aiming to walk over 4mph which is about 100 steps a minute as a minimum.

It is better to think about walking faster than the number of steps. I know the magic number is supposed to 10,000 steps a day, but one study showed older women who walked 4,400 steps a day had a lower all-cause mortality rate than those who took 2,700 – but the benefits were lost after 7,500;[286] so 10,000 would be superfluous.

Resistance Training

Once you feel you are able to walk quite a bit, you might think about incorporating some other type of exercise into your routine. The more muscle you have, the more it will protect you against insulin resistance and diabetes, no matter what you weigh. So, it would be good to incorporate some resistance training into your exercise programme. Research shows that for every 10% increase in your muscle mass to your body weight, you could expect an 11% lower risk of insulin resistance and a 12% drop in prediabetes and diabetes.[287]

Muscle is metabolically active. This means it requires fuel in the form of calories just to maintain it, even when you sit and do nothing. So, the more muscle you have, the more fat you will burn. And that is one of the reasons why men find it easier to lose weight than women – because men generally have more muscle mass than women, so they can burn fat more easily. Higher levels of the male hormone testosterone also mean that men can build muscle more easily through exercise.

Muscle takes up five times less space than fat so when you lose fat and gain muscle you will lose inches – especially around the middle of your body, which is the most toxic type of fat.

As I mentioned on page 28, muscle weighs more than fat. So, if you weigh yourself instead of measuring your body fat percentage or waist-to-hip ratio, you may get the impression that exercise is not working for you – even though it is!

Resistance training tears your muscles fibres, which then build-up as they repair, while you are resting, so it's best to avoid training the same muscle groups every day. Instead, vary the exercise groups, and give your muscles the chance to recover and repair afterwards. Focus on your upper body in one session and lower body the next so each muscle group has time to recover.

When using weights for the first time, always start with a light weight and build up slowly. The aim is to lift the weight 12 times (this is called a repetition or rep) and to do three lots of these (called sets) with one minute's rest between sets. You know you have the right weight (for now) if you can only get to eight or 10 reps in the third set. If you can do more than 12 reps in the third set, the weight is too light. You will quickly gain strength, however, so as soon as the third set becomes easier, increase the weight size or resistance.

If you join a gym, you will be given guidance on how to use the weights and the machines. Don't hesitate to ask if you are unsure. If your technique is not correct, you are unlikely to be getting the full benefit from the exercise and you could injure yourself.

Interval Training (HIIT)

You could add interval training into your exercise programme, once you feel that you are getting fitter. This is also called HIIT (high intensity interval training) and this is where you vary the intensity of your exercise within a short period of time. For instance, you could go at maximum effort on a stationary bicycle for 30 to 60 seconds and then drop down to a more comfortable level to catch your breath, before pushing yourself hard for another 30 to 60 seconds. Experts call this 'metabolic disturbance'. If you run on the treadmill for 20 minutes each time you go to the gym, your body will adapt and, over time, it will use the minimum possible energy to complete the run. It's a very clever survival mechanism, designed to avoid wasting precious resources, but you end up using less energy, burning fewer calories and losing less weight.

By using this HIIT type of exercise, your body can't adapt to the exercise and reduce how much energy it uses, and it has been shown to result in greater insulin sensitivity and better overall blood sugar control in people with type 2 diabetes than continuous activity.[288]

If you are not going to the gym, you can still use this interval training on an exercise bike at home, or in your local park where you can change the speed of your walk or run.

Other Types Of Exercise

Of course, there are other types of exercise that you might like to include such as golf, cycling, swimming and dancing. Above all, try to choose an exercise that you enjoy because you'll then be more likely to keep it up and do it regularly. It is no good signing up for a gym membership if you only go a couple of times because it is 'not your thing'.

You might enjoy yoga and tai chi and, although they won't increase your heart rate in the same way that fast walking or swimming might, they can be helpful in reducing stress and lowering cortisol. They involve slow, controlled movements with a focus on breathing correctly, which can be very calming.

Without realising it, you could have a tendency to shallow-breathe, which is effectively what happens in the fight-or-flight response, and in times of stress it can lead to hyperventilating. Yoga and other similar exercise classes can help to teach you the correct way to breathe. Yoga is also a form of resistance-training in which your own body weight provides the resistance. And both yoga[289] and tai chi[290] have been shown to help with controlling blood sugar. As a bonus, both also help with flexibility and improve the range of motion around your joints, and they can both help to improve your balance and reduce the risk of falling.

As well as these types of physical activity, there are some simple exercises you can do to improve your balance. First of all, holding on to the back of a strong chair, stand on one leg for one minute and then change sides. Repeat 10 times. Next, holding on again, roll onto your toes, count to 10, roll back on your heels, count to 10 and repeat 10 times. When these two exercises are easy to do, try using only one hand to hold on to the chair. When that becomes easy, try no hands and then eventually do the same two exercises with your eyes closed. Balancing on one leg is associated with improved cognition and a lower risk of dementia. It is hardest to do with your eyes closed, so the benefits are thought to be even greater if you can manage this.

Timing Your Exercise

Your blood glucose levels are highest 90 minutes after eating[291] and, as your muscles need glucose to exercise, it makes sense to exercise after eating in order to control your blood glucose (sugar) levels.

With type 2 diabetes you can have a much higher glucose response to a meal than people without diabetes, so it makes sense to use exercise to bring down that high response. As mentioned on page 216, 80% of the glucose uptake takes place in your muscles and without the need for insulin, so exercising after eating is an easy way to bring down a high sugar level.

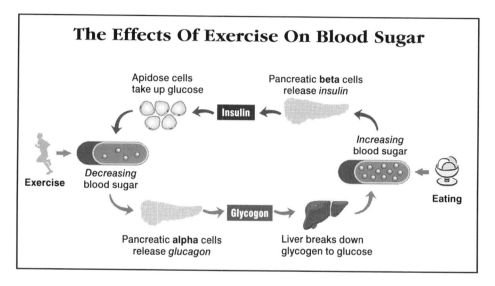

The Effects Of Exercise On Blood Sugar

Apidose cells take up glucose

Pancreatic **beta** cells release *insulin*

Insulin

Increasing blood sugar

Exercise

Decreasing blood sugar

Eating

Glycogen

Pancreatic **alpha** cells release *glucagon*

Liver breaks down glycogen to glucose

Reduce The Amount Of Time You Spend Sitting Down

As well as thinking about having structured exercise planned in your day, for example a 30-minute daily walk, also think about how long you are sitting down at one time. It is very easy to sit in front of a computer for hours, especially if you are working from home.

Sitting for too long causes your blood sugar to stay too high and just getting up and moving around between sedentary periods lowers blood sugar levels.[292]

You want to plan to break up your sitting time, so that for every 30 minutes of inactivity you take three minutes of light movement or resistance activity. Doing this has been shown to help improve reduce blood pressure in people with type 2 diabetes. [293]

An interesting study looked at breaking up prolonged sitting in overweight adults by splitting them up into three groups. One group was assigned to uninterrupted sitting for two hours, the second group to sitting with two minutes of light walking every 20 minutes over two hours, and the third group with two minutes of moderate intensity walking every 20 minutes over two hours.[294] By moving every 20 minutes, even light walking lowered HbA1c and also insulin levels.

Even if you take regular exercise, sitting for long periods of time every day can double your risk of developing type 2 diabetes.[295] Sitting down slows down your metabolism and can make you more insulin resistant; but, as you move around, your muscles work and start to contract. This helps the sugar in your blood to enter your cells to fuel your activity, and your blood sugar is reduced as a result.

Daily Movement

Think about how you can generally incorporate more movement into your daily life. It might be gardening, household tasks, getting off the bus or train a stop earlier to walk, or taking the stairs instead of the lift (elevator). All these small amounts of activity add up and make a big difference – as will having your lunch and then taking a short walk, so that your muscles can take up the glucose (sugar) from that meal. Try to do the same after your evening meal if that is possible.

Exercise Tips

- Plan your exercise session so you just do a five-minute cardio warm up before your weight training. This is a useful way to make sure you're not too tired for the weight session. You'll also burn more fat from the cardio work because all the energy in your muscles will have been used up.

- A protein-rich meal (fish, egg or pulses and seeds) eaten within half an hour of exercise will aid your muscle repair and growth.

- Don't forget to drink plenty of water – it's essential for weight loss and, if there isn't adequate water, your body will burn fat less efficiently.
- Take a break! If you don't allow your body to fully recuperate between exercise sessions, you risk losing muscle tissue and slowing down your metabolism. By letting your body recover properly with rest days you can work optimally and burn yet more fat.

To recap, exercise has so many benefits in terms of diabetes prevention and treatment by:

- Increasing your muscle mass (which, in turn, burns calories)
- Burning calories and using body fat as fuel
- Preventing and even reversing insulin resistance
- Reducing blood sugar and insulin
- Improving insulin sensitivity in skeletal muscles and fat
- Improving your body shape, reducing fat around your middle
- Reducing the negative effects of both cortisol and insulin

And for type 2 diabetes, research suggests that a combination of resistance training and aerobic (cardiovascular) exercise like walking has more impact on HbA1c levels than either of those types of exercise alone. This combination also helps to reduce waist circumference and increase fat loss.[296] But, of course, it's still just as important to include all the dietary recommendations throughout this book.[297]

PART 4

KNOW YOUR NUMBERS

CHAPTER 26:

Testing, testing…

"Over the last 30 years, increased types of nutritional tests have changed how we tailor a person's diet and supplement recommendations according to their specific deficiencies and imbalances."

Tests can be extremely useful for all aspects of your health, when you have type 2 diabetes or are at risk of it, and the range available has expanded in recent years. The following can all be extremely empowering.

Testing Whether You Have Prediabetes Or Type 2 Diabetes

This type of testing was mentioned on page 39 covering the diagnosis of prediabetes and type 2 diabetes. To recap, a blood test to assess fasting blood glucose always used to be followed by an oral glucose tolerance test, if further confirmation of the diagnosis was needed.

Once diagnosed with diabetes, then a test called HbA1c (glycosylated haemoglobin) would have been performed every few months – this gives an indication of the average blood glucose over the previous two to three months.

Now, the HbA1c test is used instead of fasting glucose to diagnose diabetes, as it is more accurate at identifying those at risk. An HbA1c level of 48mmol/mol (6.5%) or more is considered a diagnosis of diabetes.

HbA1c, glycosylated haemoglobin, is a measure of how much glucose (sugar) is attached to part of the red blood cells (the haemoglobin).

Monitoring That You Are Controlling Your Blood Sugar

It is crucial that you are controlling your blood sugar, because that way you are reducing the risk of the long-term complications explained in Chapter 5. You can monitor your level of blood glucose using a finger prick test that involves pricking your finger and dropping a small blood sample onto a test strip, which has been inserted into a monitor (called a glucometer), which analyses the blood and quickly gives you a reading. It is thought that self-monitoring of blood sugar in this way is useful in type 2 diabetes if you're using insulin or any other medication that can cause hypoglycaemia (low blood sugar) and Diabetes UK has written a Position Statement to that effect.

What is not clear, however, is whether monitoring your own blood sugar levels is helpful if you are not on insulin or a medication that can cause hypoglycaemia.

Research has suggested that 'most people with type 2 diabetes do not require self-monitoring of blood glucose and unnecessary monitoring not only wastes money but can negatively impact quality of life'.[298] And the National Institute for Health and Care Excellence (NICE) in the UK has stated that doctors should 'not routinely offer self-monitoring of blood glucose levels of adults with type 2 diabetes' except in certain circumstances – for example, for a patient who is on insulin or medication that risks causing a low blood sugar episode when they are driving or operating machinery.

But I can see how useful short-term monitoring can also be when you are changing your diet and want to see whether what you are doing is working. Monitoring also helps you check the effect that a sweetener – like maple syrup in a dessert – has on your blood sugar level. You'd then know whether you could use it or not. Monitoring your blood sugar can give you feedback to help you to know what you can manage and what you can't, and give you the confidence and motivation to carry on.

You would need to know what your baseline is before eating, so that you have a comparison, and then if you are trying something different – for example, if you have that dessert with maple syrup instead of sugar, what is your level afterwards? These monitors can be bought online and in pharmacies, and come with full instructions.

Also, as well as self-monitoring, there are ways of continuously monitoring glucose levels, with a sensor which is inserted just under the skin and measures your sugar levels 24/7, and then transmits the information to a device. This is not measuring the level of glucose in your blood, but the amount of glucose in interstitial fluid, the fluid surrounding your cells.

But, because it is not measuring what is happening in your blood, there can be differences in measurements (up to 15%) and it takes glucose up to 10 minutes to move from the blood to the interstitial fluid so there is a time lag.

It is clear that this continuous method is helpful for type 1 diabetes, but it has been suggested that it does not offer the same benefits for those with type 2 diabetes, even if they are using insulin[299] – and no long-term studies have shown that continuous glucose monitoring improves outcomes for those with type 2 diabetes.

Monitoring Your Health In The Long Term For Complications

The possible complications of type 2 diabetes are covered in Chapter 5 and it is important that you have, at least, yearly checkups. These should include a blood test to check on liver and kidney function. The same sample can check your lipid levels which would include HDL ('good' cholesterol), LDL ('bad' cholesterol) and triglycerides. HbA1c should also be included in the same blood test.

And, as inflammation is such a key factor in not only type 2 diabetes but also heart disease and Alzheimer's, it would be worth checking how much inflammation is present in your body by measuring a marker called high-sensitivity C-reactive protein through a blood test. Along with this, it would be a good idea to have your blood pressure checked and to keep an eye on your weight.

My clinic can also organise these blood tests if you have not had them in your check-ups. We use a very comprehensive fasting blood finger prick test which not only measures HbA1c but also high-sensitivity C-reactive protein, insulin, cholesterol, HDL, LDL, VLDL (very low density lipoprotein) and triglycerides. My clinic asks the lab to send you a kit and you collect the sample at home and post back to the lab. This finger prick dried blood spot test (called a Cardiometabolic Test) is much more convenient than having to go and have your blood taken from a vein. We then explain the results during a consultation. If you are interested in this test, see the Resources page 240 to contact one of my clinics www.glenvillenutrition.com.

Nutritional Tests

As well as the important medical tests mentioned above, there are some very valuable nutritional tests that you probably won't be offered by your doctor, but I think are so important for helping with type 2 diabetes.

I have mentioned both vitamin D (page 141) and omega 3 (page 118) and it is especially important to check whether you are deficient in either of these nutrients. But other nutrients such as chromium as mentioned on page 134 are also important so at my clinics, in the UK and Ireland, we also do a full blood test to check the levels of many of the important vitamins and minerals including chromium, calcium, zinc, copper, magnesium, manganese, selenium, vitamins A, C, B12, D3, E, folate, beta-carotene and the omega 6/3 ratio (see Resources page 240 for contact details). You can also just test vitamin D and omega 6/3 with finger prick blood tests, if you only want to check those nutrients, and these can be organised as a test by post through Natural Health Practice (see Resources page 240).

I think the benefits of nutritional testing are huge. Over the last 30 years, increased types of nutritional tests have changed how we individualise a person's diet and supplement recommendations according to their specific deficiencies and imbalances.

Stress Test

My clinics also offer an Adrenal Stress Test, which looks at the level of the stress hormone cortisol in your blood. The effects of cortisol remain in your body for a long time and the test is simple, safe and non-invasive – and it can determine both your cortisol and DHEA levels using four saliva samples. These can easily be collected at home or at work and sent off in the post. Your results are then explained during a consultation, alongside what action needs to be taken to correct any imbalances (see Resources page 240).

Leaky Gut Test

I talked about leaky gut earlier in the book, and it is simple to diagnose this condition with a non-invasive urine test (samples are collected at home). Two urine samples are needed. The first is a pre-test sample to give a baseline reading and the second urine sample is collected six hours after drinking a special liquid which contains two marker molecules. When the samples are analysed, the level of these marker molecules detected in the laboratory gives a strong indication as to how 'leaky' your gut is.

If the test shows you have a leaky gut, you will be given recommendations as to how to heal it back up again using natural remedies. You can then re-test the leaky gut in three month's time to make sure that it is back to normal (see Resources page 240 to organise this test).

Gut Health Test

I discussed on page 148 how important your beneficial bacteria are in helping to control your weight and reduce the risk of type 2 diabetes. These beneficial bacteria (probiotics), which live naturally in your digestive system, also have an anti-inflammatory effect on your body and are important for your general health. As I have mentioned, it is now possible with a stool test to measure your levels of beneficial bacteria and the test also shows the levels of 'negative' pathogenic bacteria and yeasts like *Candida*. The lab also checks for parasites and this is important if you have had a previous case of food poisoning and feel that your digestive function is not as it should be, as you may still have a 'bug' in there. The test also shows whether you can digest and absorb your food efficiently across fats, carbohydrates and protein.

This test is also useful if you have IBS or any digestive problems like bloating or flatulence and especially if you have had a colonoscopy and told everything is fine. A colonoscopy is important to rule out any serious problems, but it is looking more at the *structure* of your digestive system: are there any polyps for example? The digestive stool test is looking at your digestive *function*.

Any problems that are identified can be helped with dietary and supplement recommendations and then you would have a re-test a few months later to make sure that all the levels are back to normal (see Resources page 240 to organise this test).

CHAPTER 27:

Life AFTER diabetes

"If you follow the recommendations in this book – and stick to them – you could go for the rest of your life without the symptoms returning. Isn't that what you would call a cure?"

What does remission from type 2 diabetes mean – and how would you know if you are 'cured'?

This is an important question because you need to know there's a light at the end of the tunnel. And that light needs to be a long-term solution for type 2 diabetes.

Medically a 'cure' is defined as restoration to good health, while 'remission' is defined as the abatement or disappearance of the signs and symptoms of a disease. With remission, in theory, the symptoms could return. Does a remission or even a cure mean that you are not taking any medication for type 2 diabetes? What level does your HbA1c have to be? And how long should you be able to maintain this for? These are three essential questions.

In 2009, an international body of diabetes experts published a consensus paper to try and formalise what diabetes remission means. But those definitions were never formally accepted.[300] The paper stated that the mission of the American Diabetes Association is 'to prevent and cure diabetes and to improve the lives of all people affected by diabetes'.

The authors agreed on the consensus outlined below:

Partial remission = to have a level of HbA1c of less than 6.5, and a fasting glucose of 100-125mg/dl (5.6-6.9mmol/l), for at least one year with no medication.

Complete remission = to have a level of HbA1c within the normal range, and a fasting glucose level of less than 100mg/dl

(5.6mmol/l), for at least one year with no medication.

In effect, there are two aspects to remission: you will require no diabetes medication, and have normal blood sugar levels (normoglycaemia) for a year or more.

And this is doable. Obviously, the sooner you make changes the easier it will be to get your diabetes under control. If you have been told that you are prediabetic then you can reverse it.

Most of the information about type 2 diabetes says that it can't be cured. But, with the word 'cure' being defined as returning to good health, I would say that it is possible to achieve remission and get your health back at the same time.

The suggestion is that type 2 diabetes can't be cured because, even if you are not taking any medication and your blood sugar levels are healthy, it is still possible for the symptoms to return. But if you follow the recommendations in this book – and stick to them – you could go for the rest of your life without the symptoms returning. Isn't that what you would call a cure?

Yes, you are going to be more susceptible to it returning if your diet becomes unhealthy because your body has this underlying sensitivity to become insulin resistant; and you will not be able to get away with things like someone else does.

I know this doesn't seem fair, but we all have different susceptibilities and sensitivities depending on our genetic make-up and family histories. For some people it might be a higher risk of osteoporosis, cancer or heart disease. It does mean having to work harder than others to remain in good health, but the trade-off is absolutely worth it.

I do understand that it's not easy to make dramatic changes to the way you eat, particularly if you've tried diets before and they haven't seemed to work. But my approach really does work. And this is not a short-term quick fix. It is a long-term strategy to enable you to have good health going into the future.

We used to talk about lifespan, but really what you are after is healthspan. Modern medicine has increased life expectancy, but this has not necessarily come with an increased quality of life. Lifespan is the total of number of years you live. But healthspan is how many of those years you live where you remain healthy and free from disease. You are aiming to have as many years as healthy as possible.

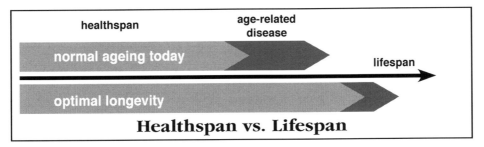

Healthspan vs. Lifespan

An example from America shows that the average lifespan is 79.3 years but if we look at the age at which someone gets a serious illness then that is their healthspan. It is interesting from the table below that type 2 diabetes occurs the second earliest, at 54 years, after chronic obstructive pulmonary disease. With respect to type 2 diabetes, this means that someone could be spending 25 years of their life on medication for type 2 diabetes and with the possible consequences as outlined in Chapter 5.

Top ten causes in the death in the US and their average or median age of first occurrence.

Disease	Deaths per Year	Age of 1st Occurance
Heart Disease	610,000	65
Lung Cancer	158,060	60
Chronic Obstructive Pulmonary Disease (COPD)	147,101	45
Stroke	140,000	65
Low Respiratory Infections	131,800	75
Alzheimer's Disease	93,541	65
Type 2 Diabetes	69,071	54
Colorectal Cancers	50,260	70
Breast Cancer	40,000	62
Prostate Cancer	25,000	66

Source: https://publichealth.wustl.edu/healthspan-is-more-important-than-lifespan-so-why-dont-more-people-know-about-it/

I would like to suggest that you think of yourself at a crossroads where one path is the road to degenerative illness, and not only type 2 diabetes but any of those listed below, in addition to ailments like arthritis where you can't move well and end up using a walking frame or wheelchair. Taking this route, you can have a long lifespan, but you don't have the healthspan that gives you energy, freedom and independence.

The other path at this crossroads takes you towards good health and I do understand it requires a bit of effort at first. You are making changes with your diet, starting a new exercise regime, improving the way that you sleep and putting new stress management strategies in place. But the benefits are enormous. You end up with not only the quantity of years ahead of you but also the quality. That is the real difference between lifespan and healthspan.

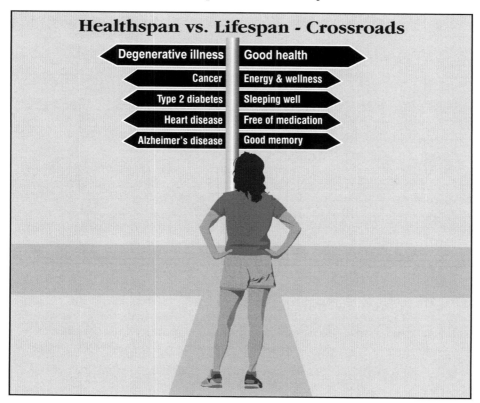

Healthspan vs. Lifespan - Crossroads

Degenerative illness	Good health
Cancer	Energy & wellness
Type 2 diabetes	Sleeping well
Heart disease	Free of medication
Alzheimer's disease	Good memory

You want to be free of medication for as long as possible, not only in terms of type 2 diabetes, but also for other chronic conditions. Age UK has pointed out that nearly two million people over the age of 65 are taking seven or more prescription medicines a day – and these put them at risk of side effects that can be severe or even life threatening. (Four million are taking at least five medicines.)

Age UK has put together a report called 'More Harm Than Good', which provides evidence that too many people are being prescribed too many drugs and there are real concerns about the possibility of unsafe combinations. They acknowledge that older people process medicines differently and they can be more susceptible to side effects such as dizziness, loss of appetite, low mood, weight loss, muscle weakness, nausea and delirium. But, as the number of medicines increases, so does the risk of falling which, of course, will often require hospital admission.

A government review in 2021 has highlighted the fact that an estimated 10% of medicines dispensed in primary care in England are inappropriate and that 15% of people are taking five or more medicines a day, with one in five hospital admissions in over 65s being caused by adverse effects of medicines.[301]

Overcoming The Barriers To Change

Making changes can be hard. But you are always more likely to succeed if you:

- Know your reasons for wanting to make a change
- Set short-term and long-term goals
- Identify your barriers
- Get support from family and friends

It takes at least three months to swap dietary and lifestyle habits that aren't doing you any good for healthier ones. Old habits are hard to change and your body and mind need that period to adjust to health-boosting changes.

- Working out what your barriers are, and how you get past them, will help you reach your weight- and shape-change goals

- Knowing what you can do when you come up against a barrier is part of the process to help you succeed in changing your habits

- It helps to not just think about the changes you want to achieve but to write them down as this makes it easier for you to be successful

Making small changes is easier

- Think about when you have tried before and didn't follow through. What held you back?

So what's stopping you? Some common barriers include:

- "I don't think I can make the changes"

- "I don't have time to do things differently"

- "I don't like healthier foods"

- "Fresh whole foods can cost more"

- "Healthy recipes can be difficult to make"

- "I want to still be able to go to the pub and have a laugh with my friends"

Be aware of the words you say to yourself: 'I can't change', 'this is too difficult'. Change your inner dialogue to be more positive. If you ask yourself questions in the negative, 'why can't I eat healthily?' your mind will provide you with negative answers that leave you trapped in a vicious cycle of failure. But if you change the wording of the question, to 'how can I eat healthily?' your mind will give you solutions and create a positive cycle of success.

Ask instead:

- "How can I make the changes?"

- "How can I make time to do things differently?"

- "What healthy foods do I like?"

- "Where can I buy affordable healthy foods?"

- "What healthy recipes would I like to try?"
- "How can I go out and enjoy myself but still stick to my new healthier habits?"

It's important to:

- Know your goals
- Plan your food changes
- Track your progress

Now think about anything that's holding you back and make a plan. Little rewards along the way can help to keep you on track.

When you've reached a sub goal (e.g. losing 7lbs or waistband is looser on you): buy a good book, scarf, lipstick or a new belt. But never reward yourself with food!

Get support. Talk to your family members and friends to see if someone wants to eat healthily with you or cheer you on. Avoid situations where you may automatically revent to your old habits:

- Change your route to work if you always passed the bakers and bought something
- If you always eat badly when you are tired make sure you get enough rest and drink enough water and this can stop a craving
- If you always feel an urge for a treat with your evening cup of tea, change to herbal tea or go and get tomorrow's packed lunch ready instead
- Think about where your 'danger points' are and work out a routine to avoid or deal with them in advance

Research shows that meal planning is an important part of keeping you on track and establishing new eating habits. Start planning your meals and snacks. Use our meal plans and recipes and your own healthy ones. If you think this is too hard or time consuming, start with a couple of days or one meal e.g. dinners for the week.

So, as the old cliché goes – today is the first day of the rest of your life. Here are my top tips to help get you started. Often the hardest part is taking the first step, but my motto is 'take the first step and keep walking'.

Getting Started

1. Don't go longer than three hours without eating.

2. Always eat breakfast, within one hour of getting up.

3. Eliminate sugar and refined carbohydrates.

4. Add protein to each meal and snack.

5. Eat essential fats.

6. Don't eat on the run.

7. Watch what you drink and have 1.5 litres of water daily.

8. Eat a wide variety of different foods.

9. Take steps to manage stress.

10. Exercise.

By taking on board the suggestions in this book you will be doing the best you possibly can to understand type 2 diabetes and how it affects you; and you will be able to manage it naturally, with nutritional solutions that will give you long-term benefits.

A good diet, regular exercise and the supplements and the herbs I recommend will, in combination, work in harmony with your body, very often achieving the same effect as drugs, but without the potentially negative side effects.

You really have got nothing to lose. The sooner you control your symptoms, the better chance you have of protecting yourself against the potentially destructive long-term damage type 2 diabetes can have on your health.

Your life, and your health, is very much in your hands.

I wish you well on your road to a healthy, happy life that is free of type 2 diabetes symptoms!

Dr Marilyn Glenville PhD

Resources

Glenville Nutrition Clinics

Consultations:

If you would like to have a consultation (either in person, on the telephone or by Zoom), then please feel free to phone my clinic for an appointment.

All the qualified nutritionists who work in my UK and Irish clinics have been trained by me in my specific approach to nutrition.

The clinics are located in:

UK - Harley Street, London and Tunbridge Wells, Kent.

To book an in-person or Zoom/phone appointment at any of these clinics, or for more information, please contact us at:

Glenville Nutrition Clinic   **Tel:** 01892 515905

14 St John's Road,   **Int. Tel:** +44 1 892 515905

Tunbridge Wells,   **Email:** reception@glenvillenutrition.com

Kent, TN4 9NP.   **Website:** www.glenvillenutrition.com

Ireland - Dublin and Galway

To book a personal or telephone appointment at any of these clinics, or for more information, please contact us at:

Tel: 01 402 0777

Website: www.glenvillenutrition.ie

Talks and Events: I frequently give talks and speak at events. See my website for my upcoming schedule: www.marilynglenville.com/events/. If you like to organise a talk near you, I would be happy to come and speak - call my clinic and ask for information about how to arrange this.

Supplements and Tests: The Natural Health Practice (NHP) is my supplier of choice for all the supplements and tests by post mentioned in this book. They only carry products that I use in my clinics and are in the correct form and use the highest quality ingredients. For more information, please contact:

Website: www.naturalhealthpractice.com
Tel: 01892 507598 | **Int. Tel:** + 44 1 892 507598

If you have enjoyed this book then please send a review.

I also invite you to join me on Facebook and Twitter for more information, tips and updates on my work.

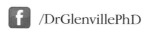 /DrGlenvillePhD

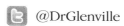 @DrGlenville

Free Health Tips

If you would like to receive my exclusive Health Tips by email, drop me a line at health@marilynglenville.com. Just mention "Free Health Tips" in the subject line and you will be added to my special list to receive regular health tips and other useful information.

Other Books By Dr Marilyn Glenville PhD

Fat around the Middle – how to lose that bulge for good

Natural Solutions for Dementia and Alzheimer's

Natural Alternatives to Sugar

Getting Pregnant Faster

Natural Solutions to the Menopause

Natural Solutions to PCOS

Natural Solutions to IBS

The Natural Health Bible for Women

Osteoporosis – how to prevent, treat and reverse

The Nutritional Health Handbook for Women

Overcoming PMS The Natural Way

Natural Alternatives to HRT

Natural Solutions to Infertility

Natural Alternatives to Dieting

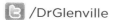 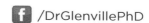

Other books by Dr Marilyn Glenville PhD

THE NATURAL HEALTH BIBLE FOR WOMEN

A practical, easy-to-use reference book guiding you step-by-step through the unique aspects of a woman's body. You will learn how nutrition, lifestyle and natural therapies can maximise your health and vitality.

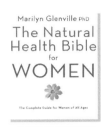

FAT AROUND THE MIDDLE

A practical action plan showing how you can get rid of that bulge once and for all.... and it's not just about diet!

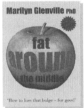

OVERCOMING PMS THE NATURAL WAY

Are you one of the 70% to 90% of women who suffer every month with premenstrual symptoms?... At last a groundbreaking approach to eliminating these symptoms for good.

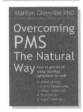

GETTING PREGNANT FASTER

Boost your fertility in just 3 months and discover the "8 steps to fertility" plan that will help you to get pregnant faster.

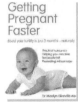

NATURAL SOLUTIONS TO PCOS

Beat PCOS and enjoy a symptom-free life, naturally. Dr Marilyn Glenville PhD has helped thousands of women overcome PCOS and now you too can benefit from her unique, nutritional programme.

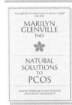

NUTRITIONAL HEALTH HANDBOOK FOR WOMEN

Everything you need to know on the most effective ways to treat all aspects of women's health - naturally.

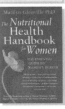

NATURAL SOLUTIONS TO IBS

How to relieve the symptoms of IBS and heal your digestive system. Full of practical nutritional advice, as well as suggestions for ways to help tackle emotional wellbeing, this brilliant book offers the vital support you need.

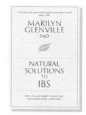

NATURAL SOLUTIONS TO MENOPAUSE

At last the definitive guide to a drug-free, symptom-free menopause and enjoying a long and healthy life beyond it.

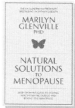

OSTEOPOROSIS - HOW TO PREVENT, TREAT AND REVERSE IT.

This ground-breaking book offers you help and advice that combines natural alternatives with conventional treatments.

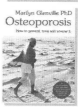

NATURAL ALTERNATIVES TO DIETING

This book will introduce you to a more natural way of eating that is satisfying and nourishing while your weight reduces naturally over time and then stabilises.

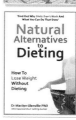

NATURAL ALTERNATIVES TO SUGAR

It's time to ditch the sugar, banish those sugar cravings once and for all and enjoy a healthy sugar-free life – and this book will show you how.

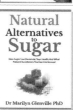

NATURAL SOLUTIONS FOR DEMENTIA AND ALZHEIMER'S

This book will help you understand the conditions and show you what you can do to protect your brain!

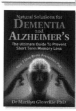

Order directly from: www.naturalhealthpractice.com
or call 01892 507598 and place your order now.

References

Introduction

1 Mainous AG *et al*, 2014, Prevalence of prediabetes in England from 2003 to 2011: population based, cross-sectional study *BMJ Open*, 4, 6

2 Ma RC *et al*, 2014, Causes of type 2 diabetes in China, *Lancet Diabetes Endocrinol*, 2, 12, 980-91

Chapter 1 – What is diabetes?

3 de la Monte SM *et al*, 2012, Dysfunctional Pro-Ceramide, ER Stress, and Insulin/IGF Signaling Networks with Progression of Alzheimer's Disease. *J Alzheimer's Dis*, 30, S217-229

4 Mayor S, Statins associated with 46% rise in type 2 diabetes risk, study shows. *BMJ*, 2015, doi: 10.1136/bmj.h1222.

5 Henriksbo BD et al, 2014, Fluvastatin causes NLRP3 inflammasome-mediated adipose insulin resistance. *Diabetes*, 63, 11, 3742-7

Chapter 2 – Diet, digestion and diabetes

6 Switzer WB *et al*, Fasting Insulin vs Hemoglobin A1c: Are We Getting It Right? *Clinical Advisor*, September 1, 2018

Chapter 3 – Understanding your risks

7 https://www.diabetes.co.uk/diabetes-and-obesity.html

8 Hill, J.O. and Bessesen, D., 2003, Editorial, *Archives of Internal Medicine*, 4, 163, 395–397

9 Dunkley AJ *et al*, 2009, Waist circumference measurement: knowledge, attitudes and barriers in patients and practitioners in a multi-ethnic population. *Family Practice*, 26(5), 365-371

10 Saad S *et al*, 2021, Abdominal visceral adipose tissue over the menopause transition and carotid atherosclerosis, *Menopause*, doi: 10.1097/GME.0000000000001755

11 Fallaize R *et al*, 2017, APOE genotype influences insulin resistance, apolipoprotein CII and CIII according to plasma fatty acid profile in the Metabolic Syndrome, *Scientific Report*, 7, 6274

12 US Preventive Services Task Force, 2021, Screening for Prediabetes and Type 2 Diabetes US Preventive Services Task Force Recommendation Statement, *JAMA*, 326(8): 736-743

13 Selvin E *et al*, 2007, Androgens and diabetes in men: results from the Third National Health and Nutrition Examination Survey (NHANES III), *Diabetes Care*, 30(2): 234-8

14 Stellato RK *et al*, 2000, Testosterone, sex hormone binding globulin and the development of type 2 diabetes in middle-aged men: prospective results from the Massachusetts Male Aging Study, *Diabetes Care*, 232, 490-94

15 Hernandez LM, Blazer DG, editors, 2006, Genes, Behavior, and the Social Environment: Moving Beyond the Nature/Nurture Debate. *National Academies Press*

16 Scott RA *et al*, 2013, The link between Family History and risk of Type 2 Diabetes is Not Explained by Anthropometric, Lifestyle or Genetic Risk Factors: the EPIC-InterAct Study, *Diabetologia*, 56(1): 60-69

17 https://www.diabetes.co.uk/diabetes-and-genetics.html

18 Rubin KH *et al*, 2017, Development and Risk Factors of Type 2 Diabetes in a Nationwide Population of Women With Polycystic Ovary Syndrome, *J Clin Endocrinol Meta*b, 102(10): 3848-3857

19 https://www.ndss.com.au/about-diabetes/resources/find-a-resource/polycystic-ovary-syndromefact- sheet/

Chapter 4 – Getting a diagnosis

20 Habib SL, Rojna, 2013, Diabetes and risk of Cancer, *Oncol*, 583786

21 De Beer JC, Liebenberg, 2014, Does cancer risk increase with HbA1c, independent of diabetes? *Br J Cancer*, 110, 9, 2361-8

22 Wang X *et al*, 2013, Inflammatory markers and risk of type 2 diabetes: a systematic review and meta-analysis, *Diabetes Care*, 36(1): 166-75

Chapter 5 – Complications

23 US Preventive Services Task Force, 2021, Screening for Prediabetes and Type 2 Diabetes US Preventive Services Task Force Recommendation Statement, *JAMA*, 326(8): 736-743

24 US Preventive Services Task Force, 2021, Screening for Prediabetes and Type 2 Diabetes US Preventive Services Task Force Recommendation Statement, *JAMA*, 326(8): 736-743

25 Noble JM *et al*, 2009, Periodontitis is associated with cognitive impairment among older adults: analysis of NHANES-III, J *Neurol Neurosurg Psychiatry*, 80(11): 1206-11

26 Dharmalingam M, Yamasandhi PG, 2018, Nonalcoholic fatty liver disease and type 2 diabetes mellitus, *Indian J Endocrinol Metal*, 22(3): 421-428

27 Roeb E, Weiskirchen R, 2021, Fructose and non-alcoholic steatohepatitis, *Front. Pharmacol.* 12:634344

Chapter 6 – Medical interventions

28 US Preventive Services Task Force, 2021, Screening for Prediabetes and Type 2 Diabetes US Preventive Services Task Force Recommendation Statement, *JAMA*, 326(8): 736-743

29 Campbell DJT *et al*, 2021, First-line pharmacotherapy for incident type 2 diabetes: Prescription patterns, adherence and associated costs, *Diabetic Medicine*, 38(9), e14622

30 de Jager J *et al*, 2010, Long term treatment with metformin in patients with type 2 diabetes and risk of vitamin B12 deficiency: randomised placebo controlled trial, *BMJ*, 340, c2181

31 Ting RZ *et al*, 2006, Risk factors of vitamin B12 deficiency in patients receiving metformin, *Arch Intern Med*, 166(18): 1975-9

32 Wilding JPH *et al*, 2021, Once weekly semaglutide in adults with overweight or obesity, *NEJM*, 3845(11): 989

33 Aroda VR, Ratner RE, 2018, Metformin and type 2 diabetes prevention, *Diabetes Spectr*, 31(4):336-342

34 Kashyap SR *et al*, 2010, Bariatric surgery for type 2 diabetes: weighing the impact for obese patients, *Cleve Clin J Med*, 77(7): 468-476

35 Cederberg H *et al*, 2015, Increased risk of diabetes with statin treatment is associated with impaired insulin sensitivity and insulin secretion: a 6 year follow-up study of the METSIM cohort, *Diabetologia*, 58, 5, 1109-7

36 Sachdeva A *et al*, 2009, Lipid levels in patients hospitalized with coronary artery disease: an analysis of 136,905 hospitalizations in Get With the Guidelines. *Am Heart J*, 57:111-1170

37 Al-Mallah MH *et al*, 2009, Low admission LDL-cholesterol is associated with increased 3-year allcause mortality in patients with non ST segment elevation myocardial infarction. *Cardiol J*, 16, 227-33

38 L Godfrey *et al*, 2014, Arginine-directed glycation and decreased HDL plasma concentration and functionality, *Nutrition & Diabetes*, 4, e134

39 Rundek T *et al*, 2004, Atorvastin decreases the coenzyme Q10 level in the blood of patients at risk of cardiovascular disease and stroke, *Arch Neurol*, 61, 6, 889-92

Chapter 7 – Eat to beat diabetes

40 Basu S *et al*, 2013, The Relationship of Sugar to Population-Level Diabetes Prevalence: An Econometric Analysis of Repeated Cross-Sectional Data. *PLoS ONE 8(2)*: e57873

41 https://www.nhs.uk/live-well/eat-well/the-eatwell-guide/

42 Lean MEJ *et al*, 2019, Durability of a primary care-led weight-management intervention for remission of type 2 diabetes: 2 year results of the DiRECT open-label, cluster-randomised trial, *Lancet Diab Endocrinol*, 7(5),: 344-355

43 Fothergill E *et al*, 2016, Persistent metabolic adaptation 6 years after 'The Biggest Loser' Competition, *Obesity (Silver Spring)*, 24(8): 1612-9

44 Finking G, Hanke H, 1997, Nikolaj Nikolajewitsch Anitschkow (1885-1964) established the cholesterol-fed rabbit as a model for atherosclerosis research, *Atherosclerosis*, 135, 1, 1-7

45 Keys A, 1970, Coronary heart disease in seven countries. I. The study program and objectives. Circulation, 41, (4 Suppl) I1-8 and Keys A, 1970, Coronary heart disease in seven countries. Summary. *Circulation*, 41, (4 Suppl), I186-95

46 https://chocolateclass.wordpress.com/2020/03/25/sugar-in-french-and-haitian-cuisines/

47 Zern TL *et al*, 2005, Grape polyphenols exert a cardioprotective effect in pre- and postmenopausal women by lowering plasma lipids and reducing oxidative stress *J Nutr*, 135, 8, 1911-7.

48 Schutte R *et al*, 2020, Drink types unmask the health risks associated with alcohol intake - Prospective evidence from the general population, *Clin Nutr*, 39(10): 3168-3174

49 Harcombe Z *et al*, 2015, Evidence from randomised controlled trials did not support the introduction of dietary fat guidelines in 1977 and 1983: a systematic review and meta-analysis, *BMJ Open Heart*, 2: doi:10.1136/openhrt-2014-000196

Chapter 8 – What's wrong with sugar?

50 Basu S *et al*, 2013, The Relationship of Sugar to Population-Level Diabetes Prevalence: An Econometric Analysis of Repeated Cross-Sectional Data. *PLoS ONE 8(2)*: e57873

51 Romaquera D, 2013, Consumption of sweet beverages and type 2 diabetes incidence in European adults: results from EPIC-InterAct, *Diabetologia*, 56, 7, 1520-30

52 Fagherazzi G *et al*, 2013, Consumption of artificially and sugar-sweetened beverages and incident type 2 diabetes in the Etude Epidémiologique auprès des femmes de la Mutuelle Générale de l'Education Nationale–European Prospective Investigation into Cancer and Nutrition cohort, *Am J Clin Nutr*, 97, 3, 571-23

53 Giovannucci E, 2005, The role of insulin resistance and hyperinsulinemia in cancer causation. *Curr Med Chem*, 5, 1, 53-60)

54 Warburg O, 1956, On the origin of cancer cells. *Science*, 123, 309-14.

55 Stocks T *et al*, 2009, Blood glucose and risk of incident and fatal cancer in the metabolic syndrome and cancer project (me-can): analysis of six prospective cohorts. *PLoS Med* 6, 12

56 Silver SA *et al*, 2005, Dietary carbohydrates and breast cancer risk: a prospective study of theroles of overall glycemic index and glycemic load, *Int J Cancer*, 114, 4, 653-8

57 Kabat *et al*, 2009, Repeated measures of serum glucose and insulin in relation to postmenopausal breast cancer. *Int J Cancer*, 125,11,2704-10

58 Walker-Samuel S *et al*, 2013, In vivo imaging of glucose uptake and metabolism in tumors.*Nat Med*, 19, 1067-1072

59 Noordam R *et al*, 2011, High serum glucose levels are associated with a higher perceived age, *Age*, 35, 1, 189-95

60 Gkogkolou P, Bohm M, Advanced glycation end products: Key players in skin aging?, *Dermatoendocrinol*, 4, 3, 259-70

61 Abate M et al, 2010, Limited joint mobility in diabetes and ageing: recent advances in pathogenesis and therapy. *Int J Immunopathol Pharmacol*, 23:997–1003.

62 Edgar L *et al*, 2021, Hyperglycaemia Induces Trained Immunity in Macrophages and Their Precursors and Promotes Atherosclerosis, *Circulation*, https://doi.org/10.1161/CIRCULATIONAHA.120.046464

63 Johnson RK *et al*, 2009, Dietary Sugars Intake and Cardiovascular Health: A Scientific Statement From the American Heart Association, *Circulation*, 120, 1011-1020

64 Shangguan S *et al*, 2021, Health Impact and Cost-Effectiveness of Achieving the National Salt and Sugar Reduction Initiative Voluntary Sugar Reduction Targets in the United States: A Micro-Simulation Study, *Circulation*, https://doi.org/10.1161/CIRCULATIONAHA.121.053678

Chapter 9 – Weaning yourself off sugar

65 Bello NT *et al*, 2011, Opioidergic consequences of dietary-induced binge eating, *Physiology and Behavior*, 104, 1, 98-104.

66 Lennerz B *et al*, 2013, Effects of dietary glycemic index on brain regions related to reward and craving in men, *Am J Clin Nutr*, 98, 3, 641-647

Chapter 10 – Sweet enough already?

67 Roeb E, Weiskirchen R, 2021, Fructose and non-alcoholic steatohepatitis, *Front. Pharmacol.* 12:634344

68 Bondonno NP *et al*, 2021, Associations between fruit intake and risk of diabetes in the Aus-Diab cohort. *J Clinic Endocrin Metab*, DOI: 10.1210/clinem/dgab335

69 Teff KL *et al*, 2009, Endocrine and metabolic effects of consuming fructose- and glucosesweetened beverages with meals in obese men and women: influence of insulin resistance on plasma triglyceride responses, *J Clin Endocrinol Metab*, 94, 5, 1562-9

70 Gepner Y *et al*, 2015, Effects of Initiating Moderate Alcohol Intake on Cardiometabolic Risk in Adults With Type 2 Diabetes: A 2-Year Randomized, Controlled Trial, *Ann Inter Med*, 163(8): 569-79

71 Schutte R *et al*, 2020, Drink types unmask the health risks associated with alcohol intake - Prospective evidence from the general population, *Clin Nutr*, 39(10): 3168-3174

72 Hill S *et al*, 2014, The effect of non-caloric sweeteners on cognition, choice and post-consumption satisfaction, *Appetite*, 83, 82-88.

73 Swithers SE, Davidson RL, 2008, A role for sweet taste: calorie predictive relations in energy regulation in rats, *Behav Neurosci*, 122, 1, 161-73

74 Feijo Fde M *et al*, 2013, Saccharin and aspartame, compared with sucrose, induce greater weight gain in adult Wistar rats, at similar total caloric intake levels, *Appetite*, 60, 1, 203-7

75 Yunker AG *et al*, 2021, Obesity and Sex-Related Associations With Differential Effects of Sucralose vs Sucrose on Appetite and Reward Processing A Randomized Crossover Trial, *JAMA Network Open*, 4(9): e2126313

76 Hazuda H *et al*, presented at the American Diabetes Association's Scientific Sessions, San Diego, 2011

77 Swithers SE, 2013, Artificial sweeteners produce the counterintuitive effect of inducing metabolic derangements, *Trends Endocrinol Metab*, 24, 9, 431-4

78 Suez J *et al*, 2014, Artificial sweeteners induce glucose intolerance by altering the gut microbiota. *Nature*, 514, 181-186

79 Diamant M *et al*, 2011, Do nutrient-gut-microbiota interactions play a role in human obesity, insulin resistance and type 2 diabetes? *Obes Rev*, 12, 4, 272-81

80 Cani PD, Delzenne NM, 2009, The role of the gut microbiota in energy metabolism and metabolic disease. *Curr Pharm Des* , 15, 13, 1546-58

81 Shil A, Chichger H, 2021, Artificial Sweeteners Negatively Regulate Pathogenic Characteristics of Two Model Gut Bacteria, E. coli and E. faecalis, *Intern J Molecular Sciences*, 22(10): 5228

82 Markus V *et al*, 2020, Anti-Quorum Sensing Activity of Stevia Extract, Stevioside, Rebaudioside A and Their Aglycon Steviol, *Molecules*, 25(22):5480

83 Bahrami M *et al*, 2009, Effects of natural honey consumption in diabetic patients: an 8-week randomized clinical trial, *Int J Food Sci Nutr*, 60(7): 618-26

84 LeBlanc WE *et al*, 2009, Formation of hydroxymethylfurfural in domestic high-fructose corn syrup and its toxicity to the honey bee (Apis mellifera), *J Agric Food Chem*, 57, 16, 7369-76

85 Makinen KK, 2016, Gastrointestinal Disturbances Associated with the Consumption of Sugar Alcohols with Special Consideration of Xylitol: Scientific Review and Instructions for Dentists and Other Health-Care Professionals, *Int J Dent*, doi: 10.1155/2016/5967907

86 Hang M *et al*, 2016, Glucitol-core containing gallotannins inhibit the formation of advanced glycation end-products mediated by their antioxidant potential, *Food Funct*, 7, 5, 2213-222

87 Li L, Seeram NP, 2011, Further investigation into maple syrup yields 3 new lignans, a new phenylpropanoid, and 26 other phytochemicals, *J Agric Food Chem*, 59, 14, 7708-16

88 Ramadan MF *et al*, 2021, Chemistry, processing, and functionality of maple food products: An updated comprehensive review, *J Food Biochem*, https://doi.org/10.1111/jfbc.13832

89 http://www.uvm.edu/~pmrc/sugarprof.pdf

90 Nagai N *et al*, 2015, Changes in plasma glucose in Otsuka Long-Evans Tokushima Fatty rats after oral administration of maple syrup, *J Oleo Science*, 64(3): 331-335

91 Scheid MM *et al*, 2014, Freeze-dried powdered yacon: effects of FOS on serum glucose, lipids and intestinal transit in the elderly. *Eur J Nutr* 53, 7, 1457-64

92 Genta S *et al*, 2009, Yacon syrup: beneficial effects on obesity and insulin resistance in humans, *Clin Nutr*, 28(2): 182-7

93 Adriano LS *et al*, 2019, Yacon syrup reduces postprandial glycemic response to breakfast: A randomized, crossover, double-blind clinical trial, *Food Res Int*, 126: 108682

94 Franchi F *et al*, 2021, Effects of D-allulose on glucose tolerance and insulin response to a standard oral sucrose load: results of a prospective, randomized, crossover study, *BMJ Open Diabetes Research and Care*, 9:e001939.

Chapter 11 – Understanding Glycaemic Index and Glycaemic Load

95 Jenkins, D.J. *et al*, 1981, Glycemic index of foods: a physiological basis for carbohydrate exchange', *Am J Clin Nutr*, 34, 362–366.

96 https://www.diabetes.co.uk/diet/glycemic-load.html

97 Brynes, A.E. *et al*, 2005, 'The beneficial effect of a diet with low glycaemic index on 24 hour glucose profiles in healthy young people assessed by continuous glucose monitoring', *Brit J Nutr*, 93, 2, 179–182.

98 Shai I *et al*, 2008, Weight loss with a low-carbohydrate, Mediterranean, or low-fat diet. *N Engl J Med*, 359, 3, 229-41.

Chapter 12 – A question of carbs

99 Swaminathan S *et al*, 2021, Associations of cereal grains intake with cardiovascular disease and mortality across 21 countries in Prospective Urban and Rural Epidemiology study: prospective cohort study, *BMJ*, 372:m4948

100 Sawicki CM *et al*, 2021, Whole- and Refined-Grain Consumption and Longitudinal Changes in Cardiometabolic Risk Factors in the Framingham Offspring Cohort, *J Nutri*, nxab177, https://doi.org/ 10.1093/jn/nxab177

101 Maruti S, *et al*, 2008, A prospective study of bowel motility and related factors on breast cancer risk, *Cancer Epid Biomarkers Prev*, 17 7, 1746-1750.

102 Feinmann R *et al*, 2015, Dietary carbohydrate restriction as the first approach in diabetes management: Critical review and evidence base, *Nutrition*, 31(1): 1-13

103 Yamada Y *et al*, 2014, A non-calorie-restricted low carbohydrate diet is effects as an alternative therapy for patients with type 2 diabetes, *Intern Med*, 53(1): 13-9

104 Goldenberg JZ *et al*, 2021, Efficacy and safety of low and very low carbohydrate diets for type 2 diabetes remission: systematic review and meta-analysis of published and unpublished randomized trial data, *BMJ*, 372:m4743

105 Tay *et al*, 2015, Comparison of low- and high- carbohydrate diets for type 2 diabetes management: a randomized trial, *Am J Clin Nutr*, 102(4): 780-90

106 Unwin D *et al*, 2021, Renal function in patients following a low carbohydrate diet for type 2 diabetes, Curr Opin Endocrin, *Diab Obes*, July doi: 10.1097/MED.0000000000000

107 World Health Organization, Joint WHO/FAO Expert Consultation "Diet, Nutrition and the Prevention of Chronic Diseases" 2003, *WHO Technical Report Series 916*

108 Vonk RJ *et al*, 2000, Digestion of so-called resistant starch sources in the human small intestines, *Am J Clin Nutr*, 72, 432-438

109 Johnson KL *et al*, 2010, Resistant starch improves insulin sensitivity in metabolic syndrome, *Diabetic Medicine*, 27, 391-397

110 Bondonno NP *et al*, 2021, Associations between fruit intake and risk of diabetes in the Aus-Diab cohort. *J Clinic Endocrin Metab*, DOI: 10.1210/clinem/dgab335

Chapter 13 – Our daily bread

111 https://www.dundee.ac.uk/stories/high-intake-dietary-fibre-and-whole-grains-associated-reducedrisk- non-communicable

112 Sandberg JC *et al*, 2017, Effects of whole grain rye, with and without resistant starch type 2 supplementation, on glucose tolerance, gut hormones, inflammation and appetite regulation in an 11-14.5 hour perspective; a randomized controlled study in healthy subjects, *Nutr J*, 16(1): 25

113 Poutanen K *et al*, 2009, Sourdough and cereal fermentation in a nutritional perspective, *Food Microbiol*, 26(7): 693-9

114 Costabile A *et al*, 2014, Effect of Breadmaking Process on *In Vitro* Gut Microbiota Parameters in Irritable Bowel Syndrome, *PLoS*, 9(10): e111225

Chapter 14 – Fat matters

115 Kavanagh *et al*, 2007, Trans fat diet induces abdominal obesity and changes in insulin sensitivity in monkeys, *Obesity*, 15, 1675-1684

116 Salmeron J *et al*, 2001, Dietary fat intake and risk of type 2 diabetes in women, *Am J Clin Nutr*, 73, 6, 1019-26

117 Ginter E, Simko V, 2016, New data on harmful effects of trans-fatty acids, *Bratisl Lek Listy*, 117(5):251-3.

118 De Roos NM *et al*, 2003, Trans fatty acids, HDL cholesterol and cardiovascular disease. Effects of dietary changes on vascular reactivity, *Eur J Med Res*, 8(8): 355-7

119 Pan A *et al*, 2011, Red meat consumption and risk of type 2 diabetes: 3 cohorts of US adults and an updated meta-analysis, *Am J Clin Nutr*, 94(4): 1088-96

120 Alvarez-Bueno C *et al*, 2019, Effects of Milk and Dairy Product Consumption on Type 2 Diabetes: Overview of Systematic Reviews and Meta-Analyses, *Adv Nutr*, 10(suppl 2): S154-163

121 Simopoulos AP, 2011, Evolutionary Aspects of Diet: The Omega-6/Omega-3 Ratio and the Brain, *Mol Neurobiol*, 44, 2, 203-15

122 Yu YH *et al*, 2011, The function of porcine PPARγ and dietary fish oil effect on the expression of lipid and glucose metabolism related genes, *J Nutr Biochem*, 22, 2, 179-86

123 Gray B *et al*, 2013, Omega-3 fatty acids: a review of the effects on adiponectin and leptin and potential implications for obesity management, *Eur J Clin Nutr*, 67, 12, 1234-42

124 Qian F *et al*, 2021, n-3 Fatty Acid Biomarkers and Incident Type 2 Diabetes: An Individual Participant- Level Pooling Project of 20 Prospective Cohort Studies, *Diabetes Care*, 44(5): 1122-1142

125 Holness MJ *et al*, 2003, Diabetogenic impact of long-chain omega-3 fatty acids on pancreatic beta-cell function and the regulation of endogenous glucose production, *Endocrinology*, 144, 9, 3958-68

126 The Preventable Causes of Death in the United States: Comparative Risk Assessment of Dietary, Lifestyle, and Metabolic Risk Factors" stud, April 2009, *PLoS Medicine*

127 McBurney MI *et al*, 2021, Using an erythrocyte fatty acid fingerprint to predict risk of all-cause mortality: the Framingham Offspring Cohort, *Amer J Clin Nutr*, https://doi.org/10.1093/ajcn/nqab195

128 Diaz-Rozzolo DA *et al*, 2021, Type 2 diabetes preventive effects with a 12-months sardine enriched diet in elderly population with prediabetes: An interventional, randomized and controlled trial, *Clinical Nutrition*, DOI: 10.1016/j.clnu.2021.03.014

129 Ponnampalam EN *et al*, 2006, Effect of feeding systems on omega-3 fatty acids, conjugated linoleic acid and trans fatty acids in Australian beef cuts: potential impact on human health, *Asia Pac J Clin Nutr*, 15, 1, 21-9

130 *de Roos NM et al*, 2003, Trans fatty acids, HDL-cholesterol, and cardiovascular disease. Effects of dietary changes on vascular reactivity, *Eur J Med Res*, 8, 8, 355-7.

Chapter 15 – Choosing an omega 3 supplement

131 Qian F et al, 2021, n-3 Fatty Acid Biomarkers and Incident Type 2 Diabetes: An Individual Participant-Level Pooling Project of 20 Prospective Cohort Studies, *Diabetes Care*, 44(5): 1122-1142

132 Ramprasath VR *et al*, 2013, Enhanced increase of omega 3 index in healthy individuals with response to 4-week n-3 fatty acid supplementation from krill oil versus fish oil. *Lipids Health Dis*, 12, 178

133 Nichols PD et al, 2014, Commentary on a trial comparing krill oil versus fish oil. *Lipids Health Dis* 13, 2

134 Salem N, Kuratko CN, 2014, A reexamination of krill oil bioavailability studies. *Lipids Health Dis*, 13, 137

135 Yurko-Mauro K *et al*, 2015, Similar eicosapentaenoic acid and docosahexaenoic acid plasma levels achieved with fish oil or krill oil in a randomized double-blind four-week bioavailability study. *Lipids in Health and Disease*, 14, 99

Chapter 16 – You are what you drink

136 Van Dam RM *et al*, 2004, Effects of coffee consumption on fasting blood glucose and insulin concentrations, *Diabetes Care*, 27(12): 2990-2992

137 Van Dieren S *et al*, 2009, Coffee and tea consumption and risk of type 2 diabetes, *Diabetologia*, 52(12): 2561-9

138 Liu F *et al*, 2015, Coffee consumption decreases risks of hepatic fibrosis and cirrhosis: a meta-analysis, *PLoS One*, 10(11): e0142457

139 Bazzano LA *et al*, 2008, Intake of fruit, vegetables and fruit juices and risk of diabetes in women, *Diabetes Care*, 31, 7, 1311-7

140 Nakamura K *et al*, 2017, Vasopressin and metabolic disorders: translation from experimental models to clinical use, *J Intern Med*, 282(4): 2980309

Chapter 17 – Know your nutrients

141 *The Independent Food Commission's Food Magazine 2005*

142 McKay JH *et al*, 2020, Overweight and obese Australian adults and micronutrients deficiency, *BMC Nutr*, 6:12

143 Yeh,G.Y. *et al*, 2003, 'Systematic review of herbs and dietary supplements for glycemic control in diabetes', *Diabetes Care*, 26, 4, 1277-1294

144 Pouteau E *et al*, 2018, Superiority of magnesium and vitamin B6 over magnesium alone on severe stress in healthy adults with low magnesemia: a randomized single-blind clinical trial, *PLoS One*, 13, 12

145 Yeh,G.Y. *et al*, 2003, 'Systematic review of herbs and dietary supplements for glycemic control in diabetes', *Diabetes Care*, 26, 4, 1277-1294).

146 Anton SD *et al*, 2008, Effects of chromium picolinate on food intake and satiety, *Diabetes Technol Ther*, 10, 5, 405-12

147 A scientific review: the role of chromium in insulin resistance, *Diabetes Educ*, Suppl 2-14

148 Singer GM, Geohas J, 2006, The effect of chromium picolinate and biotin supplementation on glycemic control in poorly controlled patients with type 2 diabetes mellitus: a placebo-controlled, double-blinded, randomised trial, *Diabetes Technol Ther*, 8, 6, 636-43

149 Yaqi T *et al*, 2013, The role of zinc in the treatment of taste disorders, *Recent Pat Food Nutri Agric*, 5, 1, 44-51

150 Chen MD *et al*, 2000, Zinc may be a mediator of leptin production in humans, *Life Sci*, 66, 22, 2143-9

151 Bo S *et al*, 2005, Gestational hyperglycemia, zinc, selenium and antioxidant vitamins, *Nutrition*, 21,186-91

152 Orhan C *et al*, 2019, Effect of supplementing chromium histidinate and picolinate complexes along with biotin on insulin sensitivity and related metabolic indices in rats fed a high-fat diet, *Food Sci Nutr*, 7, 1, 183-194

153 Rochette L *et al*, 2015, Alpha-lipoic acid: molecular mechanisms and therapeutic potential in diabetes, *Can J Physiol Pharmacol*, 93, 12, 1021-7

154 El Midaoui, A. and de Champlain, J., 2002, 'Prevention of hypertension, insulin resistance and oxidative stress by alpha-lipoic acid', *Hypertension*, 39, 2, 303–307.

155 Papanas N, Ziegler D, 2014, Efficacy of alpha-lipoic acid in diabetic neuropathy, *Expert Opin Pharmacother*, 15, 18, 2721-31

156 Mynatt RL, 2009, Carnitine and type 2 diabetes, *Diabetes Metab Res Rev*, 25(Supp 1), S45-S49)

157 Bene J *et al*, 2018, Role of carnitine and its derivatives in the development and management of type 2 diabetes, *Nutr Diabetes*, 8, 8

158 Hodgson J *et al*, 2002, Coenzyme Q10 improves blood pressure and glycaemic control: a controlled trial in subjects with type diabetes, *Eur J Clin Nutr*, 56, 11, 1137-42

159 Singh RB *et al*, 1999, Effect of hydrosoluble coenzyme Q10 on blood pressures and insulin resistance in hypertensive patients with coronary artery disease, *J Hum Hypertens*, 13, 203-208

160 Rundek T *et al*, 2004, Atorvastin decreases the coenzyme Q10 level in the blood of patients at risk of cardiovascular disease and stroke, *Arch Neurol*, 61, 6, 889-92

161 Skarlovnik A *et al*, 2014, Coenzyme Q10 supplementation decreases statin-related mild-to-moderate muscle symptoms: a randomized clinical study, *Med Sci Monit*, 20, 2183-8

162 Cederberg H *et al*, 2015, Increased risk of diabetes with statin treatment is associated with impaired insulin sensitivity and insulin secretion: a 6-year follow-up study of the METSIM cohort, *Diabetologia*, 58, 5, 1109-7

163 Pintaudi B *et al*, 2016, The effectiveness of myo-inositol an dd-chiro inositol treatment in type 2 diabetes, *Int J Endocrinol*, 913052

164 Ozturan A *et al*, 2019, Effect of inositol and its derivatives on diabetes: a systematic review, *Critical Reviews in Food Science and Nutrition*, 59, 7, 1124-1136

165 Ho Gong J *et al*, 2020, Dietary Manganese, Plasma Markers of Inflammation, and the Development of Type 2 Diabetes in Postmenopausal Women: Findings From the Women's Health Initiative, *Diabetes Care*, dc200243

166 Takaya J et al, 2004, Intracellular magnesium and insulin resistance, *Magnes Res*, 17, 2, 126-36

167 Kao WH et al, 1999, Serum and dietary magnesium and the risk for type 2 diabetes mellitus: the Atherosclerosis Risk in Communities Study, *Arch Intern Med*, 159, 18, 2151-9

168 Hruby A, Guasch-Ferre M, 2017, Magnesium intake, quality of carbohydrates and risk of type 2 diabetes: Results from three US cohorts, *Diabetes Care*, 40, 12, 1695-1702

169 Mooren FC, 2015, Magnesium and disturbances in carbohydrate metabolism, *Diabetes Obes Metab*, 17, 9, 813-23

170 Setola E *et al*, 2004, Insulin resistance and endothelial function are improved after folate and vitamin B12 therapy in patients with metabolic syndrome: relationship between homocysteine levels and hyperinsulinemia, *Eur J Endocrinol*, 151, 4, 483-9

171 Michos ED, 2009, vitamin D deficiency and the risk of incident Type 2 diabetes, *Future Cardiology J*, 5, 1, 15-8

172 Chowdhury TA *et al*, 2009, Vitamin D and Type 2 diabetes Is there a link? *Prim Care Diabetes*, 3,2, 115-6

173 Mitri J *et al*, 2011, Vitamin D and type 2 diabetes: a systematic review, *European Journal of Clinical Nutrition*, 65, 1005-1015

174 Darup D *et al*, 2012, A reverse J-shaped association of all-cause mortality with serum 25-hydroxyvitamin D in general practice: the CopD study, *J Clin Endocrinol Metab*, 97, 8, 2644-52

175 Heaney RP *et al*, 2011, Vitamin D3 is more potent than vitamin D2 in humans, *J Clin Endocrinol Metab*, 96, 3, E447-52

176 Fulghesu, A.M. *et al*, 2002, 'N-acetyl-cysteine treatment improves insulin sensitivity in women with polycystic ovary syndrome', *FerEl Steril*, 77, 6, 1128–1135.

177 Villagarcia *et al*, 2018, N-acetyl-l-cysteine treatment efficiently prevented pre-diabetes and inflamed-dysmetabolic liver development in hypothalamic obese rats, *Life Sci*, 199, 88-95

178 Dludla PV *et al*, 2018, A systematic review on the protective effect of n-acetyl cystine against diabetes-associated cardiovascular complications, *Am J Cardiovasc drugs*, 18, 4, 283-298

179 Afkhami-Ardekani M, Shojaoddiny-Ardekani A, 2007, Effect of vitamin C on blood glucose, serum lipids & serum insulin in type 2 diabetes patients, *J Med Res,* 126, 5, 471-4

180 Kook SY *et al*, 2014, High dose of vitamin C supplementation reduces amyloid plaque burden and ameliorates pathological changes in the brain of 5XFAD mice. *Cell Death Dis*, Feb 27;5:e1083

181 Johnston CS, 2005, Strategies for healthy weight loss: from vitamin C to the glycemic response, *J Am Coll Nutr*, 24(3): 158-165)

182 Palmieri C *et al*, 2006, Serum 25-hydroxyvitamin D levels in early and advanced breast cancer, *J Clin Pathol*, 59, 1334-6

183 Garland *et al*, 2006, The role of vitamin D in cancer prevention, *Am J Public Health*, 96: 252-61

184 Keum N *et al*, 2019, Vitamin D supplementation and total cancer incidence and mortality: a metaanalysis of randomized controlled trials, *Ann Oncol*, 30, 733-743.

185 Al Faraj S *et al*, 2003, Vitamin D deficiency and chronic low back pain in Saudi Arabia, *Spine*, 28, 2, 177-9

Chapter 18 – Meet your gut microbiome

186 Galland L, 2014, The gut microbiome and the brain.*J Med Food*, 12, 1261-72

187 Isolauri E, Salminen S, Probiotics: use in allergic disorders: a Nutrition, Allergy, Mucosal Immunology, and Intestinal Microbiota (NAMI) Research Group Report. *J Clin Gastroenterol*. 2008 Jul: 42 Suppl 2:S91-6)

188 Calder PC *et al*, Inflammatory disease processes and interactions with nutrition, 2009, *B J Nutr*, 101, Supp 1-45

189 DiBaise JK et al, Gut microbiota and its possible relationship with obesity. *Mayo Clin Proc*, 2008 Ar;83(4):460-9)

190 Cani PD *et al*, 2008, Role of gut microflora in the development of obesity and insulin resistance following high-fat diet feeding. *Pathol Biol (Paris)*, 56(5):305-9

191 Ridaura VK *et al*, 2013, Gut microbiota from twins discordant for obesity modulate metabolism in mice. *Science*, 341, 6150, 1241214

192 Vrieze A *et al*, 2012, Transfer of intestinal microbiota from lean donors increases insulin sensitivity in individuals with metabolic syndrome, *Gastroenterology*, 143(4): 913-6e7

193 Kootte R *et al*, 2017, Improvement of Insulin Sensitivity after Lean Donor Feces in Metabolic Syndrome Is Driven by Baseline Intestinal Microbiota Composition, *Cell Metabolism*, 26(4): 611-619

194 http://www.fao.org/docrep/007/y5609e/y5609e02.htm

195 Sonnenburg ED *et al*, 2016, Diet-induced extinction in the gut microbiota compounds over generations, *Nature*, 529(7585): 212-215

196 Robertson MD, 2020, Prebiotics and type 2 diabetes: targeting the gut microbiota for improved glycaemic control? *Practical Diabetes*, 37(4): 133-137

197 Nickerson KP *et al*, 2014, The dietary polysaccharide maltodextrin promotes Salmonella survival and mucosal colonization in mice, *PLoS One*, 9, 7

198 Anhe FF *et al*, 2020, Type 2 diabetes influences bacterial tissue compartmentalisation in human obesity, *Nature Metabolism*, 2, 233-242

Chapter 19 – Herbal help

199 Khan A *et al*, 2003, Cinnamon improves glucose and lipids of people with Type 2 diabetes, *Diabetes Care*, 26, 12, 3215-3218

200 Ranasinghe P *et al*, 2012, Efficacy and safety of 'true' cinnamon (Cinnamomum zeylanicum) as a pharmaceutical agent in diabetes: a systematic review and meta-analysis, *Diabet Med*, 29(12):1480-92

201 Ranasinghe P et al, 2013, Medicinal properties of 'true' cinnamon (Cinnamomum zeylanicum): a systematic review, *BMC Complement Altern Med*, 13:275

202 Madhavadas S, Subramanian S, 2016, Cognition enhancing effect of the aqueous extract of Cinnamomum zeylanicum on non-transgenic Alzheimer's disease rat model: Biochemical, histological, and behavioural studies, *Nutr Neurosci*, 16, 1-12

203 Wang J *et a*l, 2017, Effect of garlic supplement in the management of type 2 diabetes mellitus (T2DM): a meta-analysis of randomized controlled trials, *Food Nutr Res*, 61, 1, 1377571

204 Ashraf R *et al*, 2011, Garlic (Allium sativum) supplementation with standard antidiabetic agent provides better diabetic control in type 2 diabetes patients, *Pakistan J Pharmaceutical Sciences*, 24(4): 565-570

205 Ranade M, Mudgalkar N, 2017, A simple dietary addition of fenugreek seed leads to the reduction in blood glucose levels: A parallel group, randomized single-blind trial, *Ayu*, 38(1-2): 24-27

206 Khandouzi N *et al*, 2015, The Effects of Ginger on Fasting Blood Sugar, Hemoglobin A1c, Apolipoprotein B, Apolipoprotein A-I and Malondialdehyde in Type 2 Diabetic Patients, *Iran J Pharm Res*, 14(1): 131-140

207 Maharlouei N *et al*, 2019, The effects of ginger intake on weight loss and metabolic profiles among overweight and obese subjects: A systematic review and meta-analysis of randomized controlled trials. *Crit Rev Food Sci Nutr.* 59(11):1753-1766.

208 Zhang D *et al*, 2013, Curcumin and diabetes: A systematic review, *Evid Based Complement Alternat Med*, 636053

209 Fuangcahn A *et al*, 2011, Hypoglycemic effect of bitter melon compared with metformin in newly diagnosed type 2 diabetes patients, *J Ethnopharmacol*, 134(2): 422-8

210 Dung S *et al*, 2020, Withania somnifera (Indian ginseng) in diabetes mellitus: A systematic review and meta-analysis of scientific evidence from experimental research to clinical application, *Phytother Res*, 34(5): 1041-1059

Chapter 20 What do you eat, and *when* do you eat it?

211 Barnosky AR *et al*, 2014, Intermittent fasting vs daily calorie restriction for type 2 diabetes prevention: a review of human findings, *Transl Res*, 164(4): 302-11

212 Carter S *et al*, 2018, Effect of Intermittent Compared With Continuous Energy Restricted Diet on Glycemic Control in Patients With Type 2 Diabetes: A Randomized Noninferiority Trial. *Diab Endocrinol*, 1(3):e180756

213 Templeman I *et al*, 2021, A randomized controlled trial to isolate the effects of fasting and energy restriction on weight loss and metabolic health in lean adults, *Science Translational Medicine*, 13(598), eabd8034

214 Heilbronn LK *et al*, 2005, Glucose tolerance and skeletal muscle gene expression in response to alternative day fasting, *Obes Res*, 13(3): 574-81

215 Kumar S, Kaur G, 2013, Intermittent fasting dietary restriction regimen negatively influences reproduction in young rats: a study of hypothalamo-hypophysial-gonadal axis, *PLoS One*, 8(1): e52416

216 McCracken A *et al*, 2020, The hidden costs of dietary restriction: implications for its evolutionary and mechanistic origins, *Science Advances*, 6(8): eaay3047

217 Kim MK *et al*, 2018, Circulation, Associations of Variability in Blood Pressure, Glucose and Cholesterol Concentrations, and Body Mass Index With Mortality and Cardiovascular Outcomes in the General Population, *Circulation,* 138(23): 2627-2637

218 Chang CR *et al*, 2019, Restricting carbohydrates at breakfast is sufficient to reduce 24-hour exposure to postprandial hyperglycemia and improve glycemic variability, *Am J Clin Nutr*, 109(5): 1302-1309

219 Chenjuan GU *et al*, 2020, Metabolic effects of late dinner in healthy volunteers – a randomized crossover clinical trial, *J Clin Endo Metab*, 105(8): 2789-2802

220 https://www.eurekalert.org/pub_releases/2020-06/jhm-rnt062420.php

221 Yu JH *et al*, 2015, Evening chronotype is associated with metabolic disorders and body composition in middle-aged adults, *J Clin Endocrinol Metab*, 100(4):1494-1502)

222 Vera B *et al*, 2018, Modifiable lifestyle behaviors, but not a genetic risk score, associate with metabolic syndrome in evening chronotypes, *Sci Rep*, 8, 945)

223 Xiao Q *et al*, 2019, Meal timing and obesity: interactions with macronutrient intake and chronotype, *Int J Obes*, 43(9): 1701-1711

224 Jakubowicz D et al, 2013, High caloric intake at breakfast vs dinner differentially influences weight loss of overweight and obese women, *Obes*, 21(12): 2504-12

225 Ballon A *et al*, 2019, Breakfast skipping is associated with increased risk of type 2 diabetes among adults: a systematic review and meta-analysis of prospective cohort studies, *J Nutr*, 149(1): 106-113

226 Melkani GC, Panda S, 2017, Time-restricted feeding for prevention and treatment of cardiometabolic disorders, *J Physiol*, 595(12): 3691-3700

227 Gill S, Panda S, 2015, A smartphone app reveals erratic diurnal eating patterns in humans that can be modulated for health benefits, *Cell Metab*, 22(5): 789-98

228 Stenvers DJ et al, 2019, Circadian clocks and insulin resistance, *Nat Rev Endocrinol*, 15(2): 75-89

229 Jaeger PA, Wyss-Coray T, 2009, All-you-can-eat: autophagy in neurodegeneration and neuroprotection. *Mol Neurodegener*, 4, 16.

230 Wansink B *et al*, 2005, Super bowls: serving bowl size and food consumption, *JAMA*, 293, 14, 1727-8

231 Oldham-Cooper RE *et al*, 2011, Playing a computer game during lunch affects fullness, memory for lunch and later snack intake, *Am J Clin Nutr*, 93, 2, 308-13

232 Sierra-Johnson J *et al*, 2012, Eating meals irregularly: A novel environmental risk factor for the metabolic syndrome, *Obesity*, 16(6): 1302-1307

233 Cheng LJ *et al*, 2020, A systematic review and meta-analysis: Vinegar consumption on glycaemic control in adults with type 2 diabetes mellitus, *J Adv Nurs*, 76(2): 459-474

Chapter 21 – Carbs v ketones

234 Crosby L *et al*, 2021, Ketogenic diets and chronic disease: weighing the benefits against the risk, *Front Nutr*, https://doi.org/10.3389/fnut.2021.702802

235 Halton TL *et al*, 2008, Low-carbohydrate-diet score and risk of type 2 diabetes in women. *Am J Clin Nutr*, 87, 339–46

236 McMacken M, Shah S, 2017, A plant-based diet for the prevention and treatment of type 2 diabetes, *J Geriatr Cardiol*, 14(5): 342-354

237 Saslow LR *et al*, 2017, An Online Intervention Comparing a Very Low-Carbohydrate Ketogenic Diet and Lifestyle Recommendations Versus a Plate Method Diet in Overweight Individuals With Type 2 Diabetes: A Randomized Controlled Trial, *J Med Internet Res*, 19(2): e36

238 Goldenberg JZ *et al*, 2021, Efficacy and safety of low and very low carbohydrate diets for type 2 diabetes remission: systematic review and meta-analysis of published and unpublished randomized trial data. *BMJ*, 372:m4743. doi: 10.1136/bmj.m4743

239 Goldenberg JZ *et al*, 2021, Efficacy and safety of low and very low carbohydrate diets for type 2 diabetes remission: systematic review and meta-analysis of published and unpublished randomized trial data. *BMJ*, 372:m4743. doi: 10.1136/bmj.m4743

Chapter 23 – The role of stress

240 Shiloah E *et al*, 2003, Effect of Acute Psychotic Stress in Nondiabetic Subjects on β-Cell Function and Insulin Sensitivity, *Diabetes Care*, 26, 5, 1462-1467

241 Yun AJ, Doux JD, 2007, Unhappy meal: how our need to detect stress may have shaped our preferences for taste, *Med Hypotheses*, 69, 4, 746-5

242 Zellner DA *et al*, 2006, Food selection changes under stress, *Physiol Behav*, 87, 4, 789-93

Chapter 24 – The importance of sleep

243 Patel SR *et al*, 2006, Association between reduced sleep and weight gain in women. *Am J Epidemiol*, 164, 10, 947-54

244 Tasali E *et al*, 2008, Slow wave sleep and the risk of type 2 diabetes in humans, *Proc Natl Acad Sci*, 105, 3, 1044-9)

245 Knutson KL *et al*, 2006, Role of sleep duration and quality in the risk and severity of type 2 diabetes mellitus, *Arch Intern Med*, 166(16):1768

246 Nilsson PM *et al*, 2004, Incidence of diabetes in middle aged men is related to sleep disturbance, *Diabetes Care*, 27(10): 2464

247 Tasali E *et al*, 2008, Slow-wave sleep and the risk of type 2 diabetes in humans, *Proc Natl Acad Sci USA*, 105(3): 1044-1049

248 Gangwisch J *et al*, 2006, Short sleep duration as a risk factor of hypertension: analyses of the first National Health and Nutritional Examination Survey, *Hypertension*, 47(5):833-9

249 Daghlas I *et al*, 2019, Sleep duration and myocardial infarction, *J Am Coll Cardio*, 74(10): 1304-1314

250 Fondell E *et al*, 2011, Short natural sleep is associated with higher T cell and lower NK cell activities. *Brain Behav Immun* 25: 1367–1375, 2011.

251 Besedovsky *et al*, 2019, The sleep-immune crosstalk in health and disease, *Physiol Rev*, 99, 1325-1380

252 Cohen S *et al*, 2009, Sleep habits and susceptibility to the common cold, *JAMA Internal Med*, 169(1): 62-67

253 Spiegel K *et al*, 2002, Effect of sleep deprivation on response to immunization, *J Am Med Assoc*, 288, 12, 1471-1472

254 Rasch B, Born J, 2013, About sleep's role in memory, *Physiol Rev*, 93(2): 681-766

255 Spira AP, *et al*, 2013, Self-reported Sleep and β-Amyloid Deposition in Community-Dwelling Older Adults, *JAMA Neurol*, 70, 12, 1537-43.

256 Lee H *et al*, 2015, The effect of body posture on brain glymphatic transport, *J Neurosci*, 35, 31, 111034-44

257 Gooley JJ *et al*, 2010, Spectral responses of the human circadian system depend on the irradiance and duration of exposure to light. *Sci Transl Med*, 2, 31, 31ra33

258 Gooley JJ *et al*, 2011, Exposure to room light before bedtime suppresses melatonin onset and shortens melatonin duration in humans. *J Clin Endocrinol Metab*, 96, 3, E463-72

259 Ishihara A *et al*, 2021, Metabolic responses to polychromatic LED and OLED light at night, *Scientific Reports*, 11, 12402

260 Park YM *et al*, 2019, Association of Exposure to Artificial Light at Night While Sleeping With Risk of Obesity in Women, *JAMA Intern Med*, 179(8): 1061-1071

261 Salter S, Brownie S, 2010, Treating primary insomnia – the efficacy of valerian and hops, *Aust Fam Physician*, 39(6):433-7

262 Srivastava J *et al*, 2011, Chamomile: A herbal medicine of the past with a bright future, *Mol Med Report*, 3(6): 895-901

263 Cases J *et al*, 2011, Pilot trial of Melissa officinalis L. leaf extract in the treatment of volunteers suffering from mild to moderate anxiety disorders and sleep disturbance, *Med J Nutrition Metab*, 4(3): 211-218

264 Maroo N *et al*, 2013, Efficacy and safety of a polyherbal sedative-hypnotic formulation NSF-3 in primary insomnia in comparison to zolpidem: a randomized controlled trial, *Ind J Pharmacol*, 45(1): 34-9

265 Palmieri G *et al*, 2017, Evaluation of effectiveness and safety of a herbal compound in primary insomnia symptoms and sleep disturbance not related to medical or psychiatric causes, *Nat Sci Sleep*, 9:163-169

266 Losso JN *et al*, 2018, Pilot study of the tart cherry juice for the treatment of insomnia and investigation of mechanisms, *Am J Ther*, 25(2): e194-e201

267 Howatson G *et al*, 2012, Effect of tart cherry juice (Prunus cerasus) on melatonin levels and enhanced sleep quality, *Eur J Nutr*, 51(8): 909-16

268 Kelley DS *et al*, 2018, A review of the health benefits of cherries, *Nutrients*, 10(3): 368

269 Moloney ME *et al*, 2011, The medicalization of sleeplessness: A public health concern, *Amer J Pub Health*, 101(8): 1429-1433

270 Kripke DF *et al*, 2012, Hypnotics association with mortality or cancer: a matched cohort study, *BMJ Open*, 2:e000850

271 Karami Z *et al*, 2016, Effect of Daylight on Melatonin and Subjective General Health Factors in Elderly People. *Iran J Public Health*, 45, 5, 636-43

272 Garaulet M *et al*, 2020, Melatonin effects on glucose metabolism: time to unlock the controversy, *Trends in Endocrinol Metab*, 31, 3, 192-204

273 Lowden A *et al*, 2010, Eating and shift work – effects on habits, metabolism and performance, *Scand J Work Environ Health*, 36, 2, 150-162)

274 Gan Y *et al*, 2015, Shift work and diabetes mellitus: a meta-analysis of observational studies, *Occup Environ Med*, 72(1): 72-8

275 Folkard S, 2008, Do permanent night workers show circadian adjustment? A review based on the endogenous melatonin rhythm, *Chronobiol Int*, 25, 2, 215-24

Chapter 25 – Keeping active

276 Colberg S *et al*, 2010, Exercise and Type 2 Diabetes, The American College of Sports Medicine and the American Diabetes Association: joint position statement, *Diabetes Care*, 33(12): e147-e167

277 Kriska A M *et al*, 2021, The Impact of Physical Activity on the Prevention of Type 2 Diabetes: Evidence and Lessons Learned From the Diabetes Prevention Program, a Long-Standing Clinical Trial Incorporating Subjective and Objective Activity Measures, *Diabetes Care*, 44(1): 43-49

278 Way K *et al*, 2016, The Effect of Regular Exercise on Insulin Sensitivity in Type 2 Diabetes Mellitus: A Systematic Review and Meta-Analysis. *Diabetes Metab*, 40(4): 253-271

279 Kraemer RR *et al*, 2016, Leptin and exercise, *Exp Biol Med (Maywood)*, 227(9): 701-8

280 DeFronzo RA, Tripathy D, 2009, Skeletal muscle insulin resistance is the primary defect in type 2 diabetes, *Diabetes Care*, 32(Suppl 2): S157-S163

281 Reynolds AN, Venn BJ, 2018, The Timing of Activity after Eating Affects the Glycaemic Response of Healthy Adults: A Randomised Controlled Trial, *Nutrients*, 10(11), 1743

282 Reynolds AN *et al*, 2016, Advice to walk after meals is more effective for lowering postprandial glycaemia in type 2 diabetes mellitus than advice that does not specify timing: a randomised crossover study, *Diabetologia*, 59, 2572-2578

283 Williams PT, Thompson PD, (2013), Walking Versus Running for Hypertension, Cholesterol, and Diabetes Mellitus Risk Reduction. *Arteriosclerosis, Thrombosis and Vascular Biology*, 33(5): 1085-91

284 Colberg SR *et al*, 2016, Physical activity/exercise and diabetes: a position statement of the American Diabetes Association. *Diabetes Care*, 39(11) :2065–79

285 Yates *et al*, 2021, Obesity, walking pace and risk of severe COVID-19 and mortality: analysis of UK Biobank, *Intern J Obesity*, 45, 1155-1159

286 Lee I-M *et al*, 2019, Association of Step Volume and Intensity With All-Cause Mortality in Older Women, *JAMA*, 179(8): 1105-1112

287 Srikanthan P *et al*, 2011, Relative muscles mass is inversely associated with insulin resistance and prediabetes: Findings from the third National Health and Nutrition Examination Survey, *J Clin Endocrinol Metab*, 96(9): 2898-903

288 Jelleyman C *et al*, 2015, The effects of high-intensity interval training on glucose regulation and insulin resistance: a meta-analysis. *Obes Rev*, 16(11): 942–61

289 Innes KE *et al*, 2016, Yoga for adults with type 2 diabetes: a systematic review of controlled trials. *J Diabetes Res* 2016:6979370

290 Ahn S, Song R, 2012, Effects of tai chi exercise on glucose control, neuropathy scores, balance, and quality of life in patients with type 2 diabetes and neuropathy. *J Altern Complement Med*, 18:1172–8

291 Erickson M *et al*, 2017, Exercise after you eat: Hitting the postprandial glucose target, *Front Endocrinol*, 8, 228

292 Paing AC *et al*, 2018, The associations of sedentary time and breaks in sedentary time with 24- hour glycaemic control in type 2 diabetes, *Prev med Rep*, 12, 94-100

293 Dempsey PC *et al*, 2016, Interrupting prolonged sitting with brief bouts of light walking or simple resistance activities reduces resting blood pressure and plasma noradrenaline in type 2 diabetes, *J Hypertens*, 343(12): 2376-2382

294 Dunstan D *et al*, 2012, Breaking up prolonged sitting reduces postprandial glucose and insulin response, *Diabetes Care*, 35(5): 976-83

295 E. G. Wilmot *et al*, 2012, Sedentary time in adults and the association with diabetes, cardiovascular disease and death: systematic review and meta-analysis. *Diabetologia*, 55 (11): 2895

296 Church TS *et al*, 2010, Effects of aerobic and resistance training on hemoglobin A1c levels in patients with type 2 diabetes, *JAMA*, 304, 20, 2253-2262

297 Solomon TP *et al*, 2010, A low-glycemic index diet combined with exercise reduces insulin resistance, postprandial hyperinsulinemia, and glucose-dependent insulinotropic polypeptide responses in obese, prediabetic humans, *Am J Clin Nutr*, 92(6): 1359-68

Chapter 26 – Testing, testing…

298 Robertson SL *et al*, 2020, Continuous glucose monitoring in type 2 diabetes is not ready for widespread adoption, *Amer Family Physician*, 101(11): 646

299 Robertson SL *et al*, 2020, Continuous glucose monitoring in type 2 diabetes is not ready for widespread adoption, *Amer Family Physician*, 101(11): 646

Chapter 27 – Life AFTER diabetes

300 Buse J *et al*, 2009, How do we define cure of diabetes? *Diabetes Care*, 32(11): 2133-2135

301 https://www.gov.uk/government/publications/national-overprescribing-review-report

INDEX

glycation 39, 40, 71

glycogen 22, 23, 138, 174

glycosylated haemoglobin 39, 71, 226

goat's rue 53

good cholesterol 115, 121

green tea 199

guanidine 53

gum disease 46

gum inflammation 46

gum problems 43, 46

gut bacteria 82, 149, 150, 152, 175

gut flora 149

gut health test 230

gut microbiome 148, 176

Gymnema sylvestre 156

HbA1c 39, 40, 41, 50, 85, 138, 144, 154, 155, 157, 159, 170, 175, 207, 215, 222, 223, 226, 228, 229, 232

HDL cholesterol 16, 56, 155

headaches 19, 67, 111, 161, 175, 203, 213

healthspan 234, 235

heart attack 9, 10, 44, 48, 56, 72, 73, 143, 160, 203

heart disease 18, 21, 32, 33, 35, 36, 40, 41, 43, 44, 56, 60, 62, 63, 71, 72, 75, 98, 114, 115, 118, 119, 120, 121, 140, 168, 170, 175, 191, 210, 213, 228, 233, 234

heavy toxic metals 143

herbal medicine 52, 53

herbs 132, 133, 134, 153, 157, 206, 207, 211, 239

HFCS 78, 79, 85

high blood glucose 21, 25, 101, 129, 135

high blood pressure 18, 19, 32, 44, 129, 137, 138, 160, 168, 192

high density lipoprotein 41,

high fructose corn syrup 48, 78, 84, 85

high GI 75, 76, 91

high GL 93

High-Sensitivity C Reactive Protein 42

HIIT 219

homeopathy 212

homocysteine 140

honey 68, 84, 85, 86, 89, 90

hops 207

hormones 22, 24, 26, 31, 32, 35, 54, 79, 82, 117, 136, 169, 189, 190, 191, 192, 195, 200, 211, 213

HRT 69, 149, 151

hydrogenated fats 86

hydrogenated vegetable oil 114, 172

hypertension 195, 203

hypoglycaemia 51, 81, 162, 188, 210, 227

hypos 51

immune system 14, 46, 69, 71, 111, 148, 191, 192, 203, 215

immunity 145, 148, 154, 199

infections 37, 43, 46, 82, 192, 234

inflammation 17, 42, 46, 72, 115, 119, 145, 152, 175, 207, 228

inflammatory bowel disorders 119

inflammatory effect 118, 148

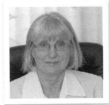

Dr Marilyn Glenville PhD

FREE Bonus Chapter

27 Mouth Watering Recipes

Many of my patients say to me that they follow all of my advice and it's been lifechanging for them to lose their symptoms and regain their health and vitality back again.

However, many of them get stuck on knowing how to put together healthy meals that are also tasty and delicious and that they can also share with family and friends.

So working together with my senior nutritionist in the clinic - Helen Ford, our resident foodie - and to help you enjoy eating your way back to good health we have put together and created this free recipe chapter for you which includes some delicious soups, appetising main meals, sauces and dressings, and mouth-watering desserts, snacks and smoothies.

Many of the recipes here are numbered and link back to the numbers in the meal planner in the book to help make it easy for you to create your meals for the day.

I do hope you find this free chapter helpful, practical, and enjoyable.

To download your easy to follow FREE bonus recipe chapter just click the link below:
www.marilynglenville.com/diabetes-recipes

Wishing you joyful cooking and the best of health

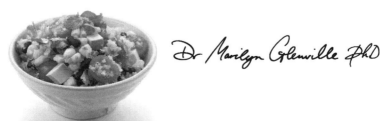

Dr Marilyn Glenville PhD